FIXING YOU®

FIXING YOU®

BACK PAIN DURING PREGNANCY

SELF-TREATMENT FOR SCIATICA,
BACK PAIN, SI JOINT OR PELVIC PAIN,
AND ADVICE FOR POSTPARTUM
ABDOMINAL STRENGTHENING.

**RICK
OLDERMAN**
MSPT, CPT

BOONE
PUBLISHING, LLC

2010 Boone Publishing, LLC

Boone Publishing, LLC

Editor: Lauren Manoy (lauren.manoy@gmail.com)
Interior Layout & Design: Lauren Manoy
Medical Illustrations: Martin Huber (mdhuber@gmail.com)
Exercise Photographs: MaryLynn Gillaspie Photography

Boone Publishing, LLC
www.BoonePublishing.com

Library of Congress Control Number: 2010920577

Library of Congress Subject Heading:
1. Backache—Physical Therapy—Treatment—Handbooks, manuals, etc. 2. Backache—Popular Works. 3. Back—Care & Hygiene—Popular Works. 4. Backache—Exercise Therapy. 5. Self-care, Health—Handbooks, manuals, etc. 6. Backache—Alternative Treatment. 7. Backache—Exercise Therapy. 8. Back ache—Prevention. I. Title: Fixing you: back pain during pregnancy. II. Olderman, Rick. III. Title.

ISBN 978-0-9821937-4-7

Printed in the United States of America

Version 1.0

ACKNOWLEDGEMENTS

In science and medicine, we build on the shoulders of those who have discovered truths before us. Writing the Fixing You series has been no different. I would like to deeply thank Dr. Shirley A. Sahrmann for her breakthrough text, *Diagnosis and Treatment of Movement Impairment Syndromes,* on which the subject of this series is based. Were it not for her textbook and seminars, which I have immensely enjoyed, I would not have been able to write the Fixing You series, much less help so many people with chronic pain or injuries. Dr. Sahrmann is a rare breed of lecturer, therapist, and researcher with a sharp mind and wit to match. Her depth of knowledge in all things musculoskeletal and biomechanical leaves me speechless.

Additionally, I would like to thank Florence Kendall, Elizabeth McCreary, and Patricia Provance for their classic text, *Muscles: Testing and Function, with Posture and Pain* (fourth edition). This book has been a tectonic plate on which our understanding of orthopedic physical therapy stands.

THANK YOU!

I would like to thank Lauren Manoy for painstakingly editing this book. She has meticulously sifted through this information and helped me strike a balance between delivering technical information and making it digestible for you, my reader.

Thank you to Michelle for being my rehabilitation model as well as a star client!

Thank you Ken Margel and Scott Sturgis for shooting the rehabilitation video for me.

Thank you MaryLynn for the wonderful photos.

Thank you to Martin Huber for the illuminating medical illustrations.

Thank you to all my patients and clients who unwittingly served as my guinea pigs and those who wittingly modeled for pictures!

Lastly, thank you to my family for putting up with long hours of writing, meetings, and physical therapy speak.

This is dedicated to Ginny.

CONTENTS

INTRODUCTION

*Thirty spokes converge upon a single hub,
it is on the hole in the center that the use
of the cart hinges.*

*We make a vessel from a lump of clay,
it is the empty space within that vessel
that makes it useful.*

*We make doors and windows for a room,
but it is these empty spaces that make
the room livable.*

*Thus, while the tangible has advantages,
it is the intangible that makes it useful.*

—LAO TZU

Fixing pelvic, back, or sciatic pain requires, among other things, an understanding of anatomy and biomechanics. That's why this book and the others in my Fixing You series presents the Fixing You approach using clear and easy-to-follow language, case studies from my practice, and pictures and diagrams to guide you, the reader, in fixing your pain. My goal is to help you visualize exactly how your body works and what's going wrong when you experience pain during your pregnancy. When you understand and can see clearly what causes your pain, you can develop and implement a plan to fix it. But knowledge is only half the answer to the problem of your pain. True healing also requires adjusting your mental processes to work for you, not against you.

Attention to your body and how it is or isn't working is absolutely necessary to recover from pain. In fact, lack of attention is a common factor in most peoples' health issues. Developing body awareness is often the most difficult—and most important—aspect of healing your pain. This is especially true when you're pregnant because your body is changing in so many ways. This book will help you understand those major changes and help you to avoid or eliminate pain during and after pregnancy.

Intention is another intangible but crucial aspect of healing. Harnessing your intention—your singular focus toward getting better—will reap enormous dividends. Visualize it, verbalize it, write it down, and live as if you are getting better every day; in the process you will discover which habits are counter to your goals. Once you identify these habits, you can change them. Each change will reinforce your intention. *Fixing You: Back Pain During Pregnancy* presents you with knowledge about the anatomy and biomechanics of back, pelvic, and sciatic pain as it relates to pregnancy; your attention and intention makes this information useful.

A TREND IN BACK PAIN

In addition to seeing clients in my private practice, corporations often ask me to help their employees with back pain. One of the ways I do this is by running back pain clinics. The back pain clinic I developed incorporates evaluating and treating volunteers from the audience with back pain to show them just how easy it is to understand the roots of their pain and fix it. This is a powerful motivator because once employees can see their colleagues fixed right in front of them, they can finally see their own light at the end of the tunnel.

After running these clinics for a while, I began to notice a trend in the women who volunteered with back pain. They all seemed to have very similar issues at the roots of their pain. It wasn't until a wave of expectant and new mothers came to me with back, pelvic, and sciatic pain that I finally put two and two together. The issues I was fixing in women who were new moms were almost identical to those I found in women in the workforce who had been pregnant years earlier. I realized the long-term significance of the toll pregnancy takes on women's bodies. For many women, pregnancy isn't just a one-shot deal. The changes that occur in their bodies sometimes never resolve—that is, until they take specific action to fix them. I began to look at women's **hip**, knee, neck, and shoulder pain through the filter of previous pregnancies. Although this book only deals with the most obvious changes during pregnancy that create pelvic and back pain, I believe many other areas of chronic pain in women's bodies can be traced back to pregnancy.

A Breakthrough

Much of the information you are about to discover is the result of my years of observing and treating patients. After experimenting with different ideas about back pain, I discovered a book that confirmed my evolving approach to diagnosis and treatment for many of my patients. Written by Dr. Shirley A. Sahrmann, a physical therapist out of Washington University in St. Louis, *Diagnosis and Treatment of Movement Impairment Syndromes* is a medical textbook that provided the missing links I had been seeking to pull together my observations. Many of the biomechanical paradigms and rehabilitative exercises in the Fixing You series have been adapted from Dr. Sahrmann's brilliant textbook. I recommend that all physical therapists purchase the book and attend her courses.

Another book I regularly reference is Florence Kendall, Elizabeth McCreary, and Patricia Provance's classic, *Muscles: Testing and Function, with Posture and Pain*. This textbook is a wealth of information for understanding precise musculoskeletal anatomy and testing. It is a standard in physical therapy, and I regularly refer to it for isolating muscle testing. It guides me in specifically analyzing and thinking creatively about function. By understanding muscle function on a basic level, I can better hypothesize functional deficits that may be occurring at a systemic level.

But this book is written for you, the expectant or new mother, to guide you in healing yourself. I've simplified and distilled my medical training to reflect the majority of problems I've found when treating back or pelvic pain in women just like you. I've prioritized the corrective exercises I've found most powerful for your condition. I've bolded vocabulary words and added information boxes to help clarify words or concepts. I've also created videos of all the exercises and tests to enhance the effectiveness of your program. To access these free video clips, visit my website **www.FixingYou.net**. Type in the code at the end of this book to access the extra material.

HOLISTIC FUNCTION

Your body is the sum of individual units working together to create functional movement. Bones, muscles, tendons, nerves, and ligaments can all be addressed individually, but it's important to understand how these structures work collectively to fulfill a purpose: pain-free movement of the body. So, while it's imperative that individual "chinks in the armor" are found and corrected, visualizing how the whole works together is just as important.

This concept also works from the other direction; training movement and/or function reinforces and assists in correcting individual muscles' poor performance. In this book, I've introduced the key individual players—the parts that make up the whole—and also shown how they play together to create function, much like a symphony. You are responsible for bringing them in line to create your concert.

I wish you the best in your pursuit for solutions to your pain. You are not alone in your search for answers. I truly believe that with a little thought and effort on your part, the Fixing You approach will help you fix your pain, as it has for my clients.

The beauty of the body is that results happen quickly when you are doing the right thing. Most of my clients feel significantly better after only one or two treatments. Often, they understand they are on the right path within minutes of performing an exercise. Emboldened by this sense, they become more committed to the process of fixing themselves. You can have the same feeling of empowerment. There is no magical technique or device that will fix you. Only you can fix you—so let's get started on giving you the tools to do just that.

1 | MINDFUL HEALING

There is not a single problem in LIFE *you cannot* RESOLVE, *provided you first solve it in your* INNER WORLD, *its place of origin.*

—PARAMAHANSA YOGANANDA

The most powerful aspect of the Fixing You approach is that it shows you what's wrong, actually gets you to feel that certain muscles or movements aren't working and how your body feels better when they are corrected. This helps define the problem. It gives issues a beginning and an end, allowing you to compartmentalize pain—and therefore see when and how the solution will happen. Given the tools to understand and correct your back, sciatic, or pelvic pain, I hope you will feel a sense of empowerment that will motivate you to work harder to fix yourself. If you can define an issue, then you have the power to fix it—and that motivation will get you results.

Even though the exercises in this book aren't "fitness" exercises per se, the concepts behind them are useful for and relevant to a fitness standpoint. It's best to begin an exercise program early in your pregnancy—the earlier, the better, especially if you weren't regularly exercising prior to getting pregnant and have decided to turn over a new leaf. Although the corrective exercises I present in this book are gentle, it's always best to check with your physician prior to beginning a new exercise routine. Bring this book to your next appointment and show it to your doctor, so he or she can get a feel for the principles behind the exercises and see the pictures and descriptions. This ensures that everyone is on the same page, so to speak. Make sure you contact your physician ahead of time to let him or her in on your plans.

Regardless, getting your head into your plan is essential. Without your commitment, it will never get done. The exercises and techniques I describe in this book will only help you if you commit to them—or more important, if you commit to yourself. In my experience, there are three processes involved with fixing pain: You have to visualize the problem and the change needed to solve it, verbalize your intention and write down a plan of action to fix it, and take action to implement your plan.

> Creating **positive change** involves internalizing your desire, verbalizing your intention, and acting on it.

VISUALIZE THE PROBLEM

The information in this book will help you "see" what's at the bottom of your back or pelvic pain and how to fix it by giving you a glimpse into your underlying anatomy. You'll notice that as much as I discuss the anatomy of a problem, I also talk about movement. There's little use in learning anatomy if you don't also understand how it creates movement. You'll learn what happens to your joints if your muscles aren't working correctly and how that causes pain.

> Set aside 10 seconds throughout the day to **get in touch** with your body and visualize its muscles.

In most cases, back pain in new or expectant mothers is the result of the changes to the shape of their bodies; those changes consequently alter their movement patterns. This speaks to what I describe as the chronic pain cycle (Figure 1.1). Changes in muscles, joint motions, and movement habits are interrelated, reinforcing each other and your pain. Anatomical changes in muscles create biomechanical changes in how the joints move. These biomechanical changes alter the way you move, which creates poor movement habits called movement dysfunctions; movement dysfunctions then reinforce the original anatomical and biomechanical changes.

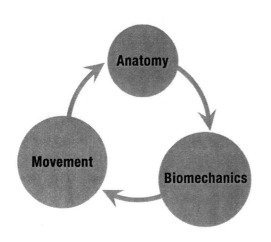

Chronic Pain Cycle

Figure 1.1 Fixing pain involves correcting each part of the pain cycle.

This book will help you visualize these changes and teach you how to offset them as best you can. There are ample illustrations and pictures that highlight key concepts for you, so you'll know exactly what's happening to your body and how these changes can continue to affect your body after pregnancy. Look at the illustrations of key muscles in this book, and take some time to visualize where they are on your body and what they do. Use your fingers to feel the area in question to help yourself consciously connect with it.

VERBALIZE YOUR INTENTION

Solidify your ideas and support your intention to heal by talking to friends or family or writing down your plan. Often, discussing plans brings their fruition one step closer. Now that you're pregnant or a new mom with lots to juggle every day, you may feel like it's too much to handle, but you'll soon see how simple it will be to get rid of your pain.

I think all of us have had a time in our lives when we secretly challenged ourselves to reach a goal but didn't tell anyone about it because saying it would heap more responsibility on our shoulders to make it come true. Commit to yourself by telling your friends and family about your goals. By telling them that you believe you will become pain free, you have already made a shift in your consciousness to make it happen. Say it! Write it down! Announcing it isn't a leap of faith, it's an affirmation of your future.

"Right," you're saying, "I'll just squeeze that in between work, appointments with the doctor, shopping for the baby, eating right, resting, reading all the books and magazines I've bought, and keeping my head screwed on straight." Well, yes, because pain distracts you from all these other important things in your life. Keep a few simple notes that describe what reduces your pain and areas you still need help in. This reinforces that you're in control of what's happening to and around you.

Take Action to Implement Your Plan

Finally, you must take action to eliminate your pain. I guarantee that if you don't take action, your goals won't materialize. I often initially hear frustration and resignation from my postpartum clients that their bodies will never be the same. Your body won't be the same; it will be better because you'll have strength, knowledge, and awareness you've never had before. There's nothing more satisfying than seeing a client brighten after having cleared a hurdle to her goal of regaining her body and her life. You may have to set aside time for several exercise sessions each day until the length or strength of the involved muscles is at least partially corrected. Once this is accomplished, your pain will diminish, and you can begin whittling down the exercises.

> Physical therapists use **short- and long-term goals** to create our treatment plans—and you should do the same.

A maintenance plan is often necessary because the effects of pregnancy don't just vanish once your baby is born. You'll have to reeducate your body and keep it from slipping back into poor habits or postures. You must feel and notice how your body is moving and performing during the day and when exercising. Attending to your specific mechanics will deliver results. I see it all the time, and your body is built no differently than all the other women this approach has worked for.

It's easy to get down on yourself for not being in the shape you want to be in; that's why short- and long-term goals are helpful. They keep you on track, and they prevent you from berating yourself for not being further along.

Goals should be realistic and as specific as possible to be helpful. For instance, a short-term goal while pregnant could be to perform four, five-minute sessions each day during the next four weeks to eliminate your pain. A short-term goal postpartum could be to set aside five, two-minute sessions each day for three weeks to practice activating your abdominal muscles (try the Heel Slides or Knee Wobbles exercises on pages 82 and 84).

Long-term goals should also be specific; for instance, set a goal that in five weeks you'll maintain two, three-minute corrective exercise sessions each day to keep your pain at bay. A long-term postpartum goal could be that in six weeks, you'll be able to keep your lumbar spine flat while you perform 15 Heel Slides on each leg.

With the demands of our busy days, it can be difficult to stay focused on making changes to established habits or patterns. That's why I recommend you set up a way to remind yourself of your new goals and to check in on your habits. Wear a special bracelet, ring, string, or rubber band around your wrist to remind you of the changes you're evoking in your mind and body. Place stickers on the dashboard of your car, the clock, your watch, your telephone—anything you use or look at frequently—to remind yourself that you're getting better every day by correcting those habits that feed your pain.

Slow down and feel what your body is telling you when performing the tests and corrective exercises and when you're out and about during the day.

My hope is that with the guidance of this book, you will be vigilant in taking care of yourself during pregnancy to prevent back, pelvic, or sciatic pain. If you already have those issues, then the exercises in Section 3 will fix them. Taking care of your body after pregnancy is just as important. Even if you didn't suffer from any of these aches and pains, your body has been altered from the experience of bringing your baby to term. Take some time to discover these changes. It will have an enormous payoff in the future by preventing back, sciatic, or pelvic pain.

People often believe they'll have to set aside a lot of time to fix their pain. Not true. Each session should take no longer than three to five minutes, two to five times each day. In total, I am asking you to take a maximum of 25 minutes a day to get rid of your pain. Chances are that you won't need nearly that much time. That doesn't sound too bad, does it?

Visualizing, verbalizing, and taking action to stop your pain must happen now. You will see that you can easily eliminate your pain but also that no one else can do this for you. You must do it for yourself. I know at this point you feel it will be an almost insurmountable mountain for you to climb, but you'll soon find it's only a rolling hill. You have in your hands the perfect tool to help you understand why you have pain and how to fix it. Don't be surprised if it is diminished or completely gone after the first exercise session. The body responds quickly to those things that are good for it. Now you'll learn just what those things are.

On this note, I'd like to add a word of caution. There are many possible causes of pelvic or back pain while pregnant. Therefore you should first consult your physician to rule out other diagnoses. Once you both are sure the pain must be musculoskeletal in origin, then you can begin using the concepts in this book to fix it. Good luck!

2 | UNDERSTANDING YOUR ANATOMY

KNOWLEDGE *of any kind gets metabolized spontaneously and brings about a* **CHANGE** *in* **AWARENESS** *from where it is possible to create* **NEW REALITIES.**

—**DEEPAK CHOPRA**

Research shows that staying fit during pregnancy is not only good for the mother but also for the baby. During this time it's even more important not to let pain interfere with your exercise routine, much less your general state of well-being. Many would-be mothers resolve to accept back, pelvic, or sciatic pain as a rite of passage, but this need not be the case. The first step in fixing a problem is defining the issue. As you will soon learn, fixing back, pelvic, or sciatic pain can be a relatively simple process once you understand the key parts of the equation and how to improve their function.

Even if you don't have back pain now, I believe pregnancy can contribute to back, neck, hip, or knee pain later in life. The metamorphosis of a mother's body during pregnancy creates strength and range-of-motion deficits that are at the root of many chronic injuries. Often these changes don't immediately manifest as pain but instead lay the foundation for injury later in life.

Back pain during pregnancy is caused by adaptations your body makes as the fetus grows. Some of your ligaments and muscles stretch while others tighten. Even your spine changes shape. You won't sense these changes because they happen gradually. You are about to learn exactly what these changes are and how to fix them. This will also help you bounce back faster after your baby is born because you'll understand exactly how your body has changed and how to safely resume exercising. Knowing about these changes will give you the power to reverse them, stave off future injury, and help you get your old shape back sooner once your baby is born!

Many of you will be tempted to skip forward to Section 3: Corrective Exercises to immediately begin fixing your body and reducing pain. That's fine, although I highly recommend reading through the entire book first so you understand more completely why you have pain and what you may be doing that exacerbates it. It's important to understand that what you do throughout the day can either contribute to your pain or help relieve it. In addition to the specific exercises, it's critical to become aware of and modify any pain-causing habits. Changing unhealthy habits is a long-term solution that will eliminate your pain for good, and this book will help guide you in that process.

Congratulations and good luck!

THE ROOTS OF BACK PAIN DURING PREGNANCY

Being pregnant is a magical time for most women. However, it can also wreak havoc on your body. Of course, we'd like to avoid that, so let's begin with some basic anatomy so you'll understand how everything fits together. There are three areas we're primarily concerned with: The first is your spine. This is influenced in large part by the second area, your **pelvis**. The third element is your **abdominal muscles**. You'll also learn what happens to your joints if your muscles aren't working correctly and how that causes pain. Finally, we'll put all the elements together to understand how these changes create painful movement habits that reinforce your problems in each of the areas above.

While reading this book, keep in mind that these three areas are related in terms of function. Each affects the other. To fix your pain, recover from your pregnancy, or prevent future injury, you'll have to learn about and fix these potential problems. Don't worry though, it's easier than you think!

Looking Closely at Your Spine

To understand why you have back or sciatic pain, it's important to first understand how the spine is shaped and how it moves. This may seem elementary, but bear with me; you'll get the big picture in just a moment.

Looking at the spine from the side, you'll see it's curvy. The neck (cervical) area has an inward (lordotic) curve that reverses to an outward (kyphotic) curve just below it in the upper trunk (thoracic) region. Moving further down, we see another lordotic curve in the lower back (lumbar) area (Figure 2.1, page 26). These curves are important in allowing the spine to move well. When they change, your back moves differently, which causes pain.

Now let's look at how the back moves. The spine needs to perform four movements well to be pain free. The first movement is **flexing** (bending forward), such as when we bend down to pick up an object off the floor. When we bend down, the lumbar curve reduces, or flattens out, a bit.

The second movement is **extending**, or straightening back up. After we pick up that object, we need to stand up tall again, which the spine does by extending. This restores the lumbar curve back to normal from its flexed, flattened position.

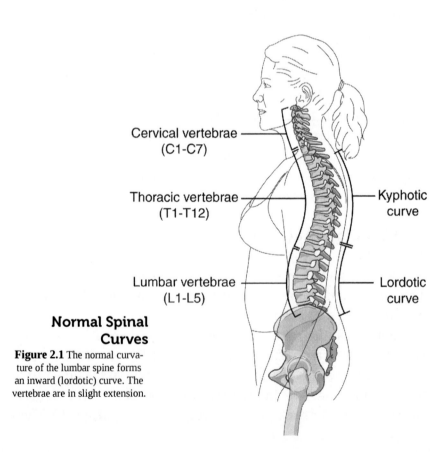

Cervical vertebrae
(C1-C7)

Thoracic vertebrae
(T1-T12)

Kyphotic
curve

Lumbar vertebrae
(L1-L5)

Lordotic
curve

Normal Spinal Curves

Figure 2.1 The normal curvature of the lumbar spine forms an inward (lordotic) curve. The vertebrae are in slight extension.

The third movement is **side-bending**. For instance, if you're sitting at your desk and need to pick up an object beside you on the floor, you'll side-bend to pick it up and then side-bend in the opposite direction to come back up and place it on your desk.

The last movement our spine needs to do well is rotate, such as when twisting around to see what just fell on the floor. Just about every activity or sport we engage in involves **rotation**. Side-bending and rotation are interrelated: When we side-bend, our **vertebrae** also rotate in the opposite direction. So if you reach down to your left side, your spine will consequently rotate to the right. I'm all about simplifying things, so let's combine side-bending and rotation and just call it "rotation."

So after all is said and done, we can say that for the spine to be happy, it needs to adequately flex forward, extend backward, and rotate to either side.

Now that we've seen what the curves of a spine are supposed to look like and how the spine is supposed to move, let's put these ideas together. Remember the lordotic curve of the lower spine? Well, the reason it has a lordotic curve is because the lumbar vertebrae are in some **extension** (arching backward; see Figure 2.1 on the opposite page). If you can understand this, then you are well on your way to understanding why women develop back or sciatic pain during pregnancy.

As the fetus develops, your belly grows farther out in front of you. To avoid tipping over onto your face, your spine must extend backward to counter this new development. Therefore, the lordotic curve of your spine

> Even though **sciatic pain** has its roots in spine function, it can also result from poor pelvic positioning because the **pelvis controls the spine**.

becomes more pronounced (Figure 2.2, page 28). This increased lordotic curve then changes how the spine bends forward. Now, because of its new shape, the vertebrae don't get to flex as much as they used to when bending forward; instead, they remain in some extension. Also, when you return from bending forward, your spine starts out in a more extended position and moves into even further extension while resuming its new, larger lordotic curve. So, the increased weight in your tummy has caused your lumbar spine to increase its lordotic curve, which then alters how you bend forward and straighten back up.

When the spine assumes an extension posture, as in Figure 2.8 (page 35), it becomes more difficult for the vertebrae to recover their normal lordotic curve. Pain can result from this abnormal stress to the spine and surrounding tissues. This is what I refer to as an **extension problem**, meaning the spine is either extended too much, it's unable to flex well, or the abdominal muscles lack the necessary strength to stabilize the spine against extension-producing stresses (i.e., those created from an **anteriorly** tilted

Anterior Pelvic Tilt

Figure 2.2 During the later stages of pregnancy, the pelvis tilts forward (anterior pelvic tilt), which increases the lordotic curve of the lumbar spine.

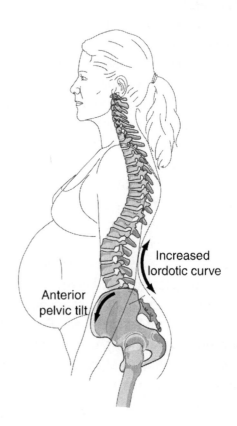

Increased lordotic curve

Anterior pelvic tilt

pelvis, which we'll discuss in just a moment). Excessive spinal extension manifests not only as back pain but also as sciatic pain. Because the **sciatic nerve** is composed of nerve roots that exit from the lumbar spine, restoring its normal curve fixes sciatic pain.

Aside from extension problems, the spine can also become rotated. I call this a **rotation problem**. Rotation problems can exacerbate back pain due to extension problems. I typically address the extension problem first because that is usually the primary irritant to the back. If pain remains, then we look into correcting the rotation problem. This usually involves identifying and correcting habits that hold the spine in prolonged patterns of side-bending or rotation.

For instance, sitting there reading this book, you may have one leg folded underneath you, or you may be leaning on a pillow to your left. Maybe your desk is organized so the items you most frequently use are located to the right, which requires you to rotate to the right more often than to the left. Over time, the spine permanently adopts these rotated positions, which can cause back pain. Still with me? Good! Let's now move on to the pelvis and see how changes there affect the spine.

Looking Closely at Your Pelvis

The pelvis is one of the key players in fixing back pain or sciatica during pregnancy. The pelvis is the keystone to a healthy spine. If it's sitting pretty, then our spine usually is too. That is because the spine is stacked right on top of the pelvis.

The pelvis is made up of three bones (okay, technically there are more than three, but we'll keep it simple for our purposes): the **sacrum** and two **ilia**. The sacrum is the part of the pelvis that forms a joint with the lowest **lumbar vertebra**. This joint is called the lumbosacral junction. It's here that most spinal movement happens when we bend forward and straighten back up. This is important to keep in mind because pain in the body typically happens at joints that move too much rather than those that move too little. Therefore where the spine meets the pelvis, the lumbosacral junction, is more susceptible to injury than other areas of the spine.

The sacrum also forms a joint with the ilia that flank it on either side (see Figure 2.3). This is the SI joint (sacro-iliac joint), which many of you have probably heard about online or from health care providers. This joint normally doesn't move that much, but it may be more mobile during pregnancy. This is because the pelvis widens in preparation for the birth of your baby. This widening is helped by a hormone called **relaxin** that may help loosen pelvic joints, including the SI joints. Therefore they'll move more than usual, especially during the last trimester.

The Pelvis

Figure 2.3 The pelvis is composed of a sacrum and two ilia. Each ilium has a socket with which the thigh bone interacts to form the hip joint. The sacrum also forms a joint with the lowest lumbar vertebra (lumbosacral junction).

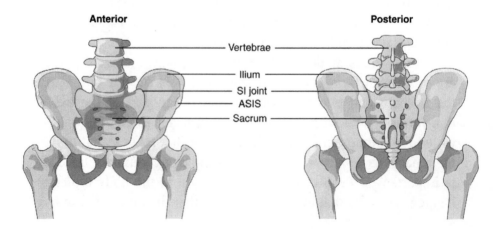

The ilia are irregularly shaped bones that contain sockets into which the head of the thigh bone (femur) inserts to form the hip joint. The muscles that attach to the ilia determine how the whole pelvis functions. So here's the big picture: The way the pelvis rests and moves guides how well the spine works because the two are literally linked together. Let's look at this a little more closely.

A pelvis in a good resting position isn't tilted too far forward or too far backward (see Figure 2.4). When the pelvis is in its ideal resting position, there is a slight inward curve of the lumbar spine, a normal lordotic curve. Remember, a normal lordotic curve helps your spine bend and straighten well (which you'll be doing a lot of once the baby is born!).

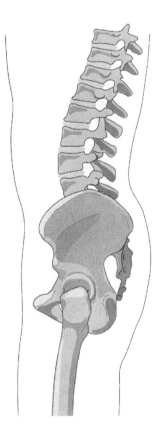

Neutral Pelvis
Figure 2.4 A neutral pelvis helps the spine maintain a normal lordotic curve.

To learn more about **flexion problems** or back pain in general, read **Fixing You: Back Pain.**

Changes in the way the pelvis rests or moves affect the lordotic curve and can strain the lumbosacral junction. For instance, if the pelvis is slightly tilted back, as in a **posterior pelvic tilt**, it tends to reduce or flatten the lordotic curve (see Figure 2.5). This means the spine is in a permanent state of slight **flexion**, although it should ideally be in a little extension. A flattened spine at rest is more likely to flex too much, too soon, or too easily when

Posterior Pelvic Tilt

Figure 2.5 A posterior pelvic tilt flattens the lumbar spine, reducing the lordotic curve.

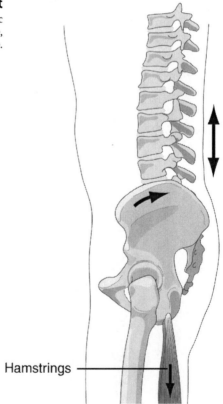

Hamstrings

bending over. A spine with this tendency is said to have **flexion problems**. You've probably already figured out this is an unlikely scenario in pregnant women because of the way the spine changes as the fetus grows.

In fact, exactly the opposite happens as you move into the later months of pregnancy. The weight of the fetus gradually causes your pelvis to tilt forward into a position called **anterior pelvic tilt** (Figure 2.6).

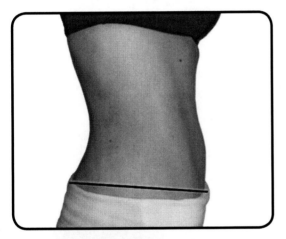

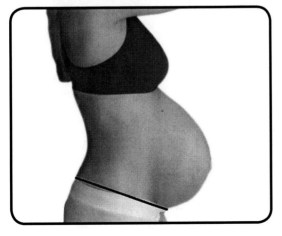

Changes in Pelvic Tilt During Pregnancy

Figure 2.6 The straight lines depict the orientation of the pelvis. The first picture shows a relatively neutral pelvis. Notice the change in the orientation of this same woman's pelvis in the second picture taken during her third trimester. It is tilted forward (anteriorly) in response to the added weight she is carrying in front.

Over time, an anterior pelvic tilt will cause the muscles in the front of the pelvis (the tensor fascia lata [TFL], rectus femoris, and sartorius) to shorten; the shortened muscles then reinforce the anterior pelvic tilt. It's really a chicken-and-egg situation. This pelvic tilt also causes the spine's lordotic curve to increase (Figure 2.7).

Anterior Pelvic Tilt

Figure 2.7 Muscles attaching to the front of the pelvis, including the tensor fascia lata (TFL) and rectus femoris, can become tight; this contributes to anterior pelvic tilt and a greater lordotic curve (spinal extension).

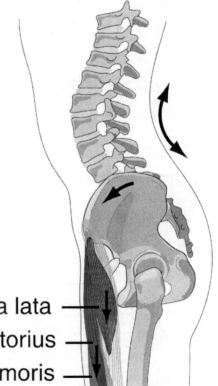

Tensor fascia lata

Sartorius

Rectus femoris

Remember, a lordotic curve means the lumbar vertebrae must be slightly extended, so a bigger lordotic curve means even more spinal extension. When you think about it, your spine really is bending backwards to offset the growing fetus's weight that's pulling you forward (Figure 2.8). This happens gradually as the pregnancy progresses and is largely ignored. The problem is that it happens at the vertebral segments that move the most—usually those at the lumbosacral junction or a level or two above it.

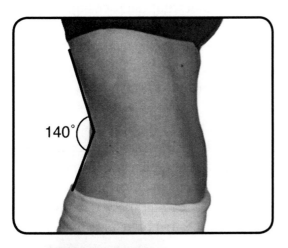

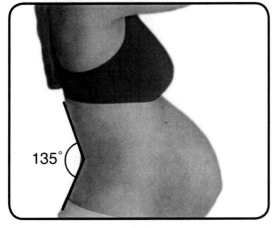

Increased Angle of Lumbar Lordosis

Figure 2.8 During pregnancy, the lordotic curve of the lumbar spine becomes more pronounced, which leads to back pain or sciatica. Even a small degree of change can lead to abnormal tissue stress.

It's important to understand that the pelvis can develop an anterior tilt even if the muscles in the front of the pelvis don't tighten up. In about 10 percent of people I treat, I've seen the pelvis just "fall" into an anterior tilt due to poor abdominal control and perhaps lumbar spine hypermobility. Unfortunately, these people can't rely on the TFL & Quadriceps Stretch (page 72) to help them because those muscles aren't tight. Instead, they must focus on strengthening the abdominals to hold the pelvis and spine in a better position. This should be strongly reinforced by monitoring and changing daily habits that tend to pull the pelvis into an anterior tilt, such as standing with "locked" knees.

Set up a reminder such as stickers or wearing special jewelry to help remind you to check in on and **change poor habits** that contribute to pain.

Standing with straightened, or locked, knees pitches the pelvis into an anterior pelvic tilt. You've learned that this posture promotes further back extension, in the form of an increased lumbar **lordosis**, which causes back pain. Regardless of whether the muscles in front of your pelvis are tight or not, changing this habit will have a dramatic effect on reducing your back pain. Because it is such a common habit, I recommend that you use a reminder such as a string around your finger or wrist to remind you to unlock your knees whenever possible.

Looking Closely at Your Joints

I've mentioned a couple times that problems arise from joints that move too much, so let's discuss that further. Sites of excessive joint movement, or hypermobility, are where pain most often occurs. Lack of joint movement, or hypomobility, usually creates hypermobility at the joints above or below it. Your body will get the job done as best it can, and if a joint isn't moving enough (**hypomobile**), the other joints around it have to make up for that deficit by moving too much. During pregnancy, the vertebrae of the lower spine become **hypermobile** due to several factors: (1) increased weight in the front of the stomach pulling the spine into more extension; (2) an anteriorly tilted pelvis; (3) pelvic muscles that become too tight; and finally, (4) elevated production of the hormone relaxin. These factors in combination create a perfect storm for back, pelvic, or sciatic pain.

> Pain is usually due to **joint hypermobility**. It's much like repeatedly bending a copper pipe. A crease will eventually form at the point that bends the most. It is at this point the pipe will break.

For these reasons, increased spinal extension is actually at the root of most back pain during pregnancy. For many women, the seeds of future back injury are planted at this time unless care is taken to reverse these anatomical changes after the baby is born.

Client Connection:
Dawn's Extension & Rotation Problem

I recently worked with Dawn, a friend who was in her sixth month of pregnancy and complained of sciatic and lower back pain. She was young, healthy, and fit, and she went on frequent walks in the foothills of the Rocky Mountains. Her sciatic pain was a new issue, and it seemed worse in the morning. So I visited her house to see what I could do. While our kids played, I quickly assessed her problem.

I found that her lumbar spine was arching (extending) too much, and she also had a rotated pelvis. Because her pain was worse in the morning, I assessed her sleeping posture. I found that her spine was rotated and extended while sleeping, which caused her to experience more pain in the morning.

The Fixing You Approach for
Extension & Rotation Problems

I gave Dawn two recommendations. The first was to lie on a folded towel when she was on her side. This removed side-bending stress to her spine. Remember that when the spine side-bends, it also rotates to the opposite direction. The folded towel prevented side-bending and therefore rotation, which relieved stress to her spine and sciatic nerve while she slept.

The second recommendation was to practice flexing her spine (reducing the lordotic curve) throughout the day; the repeated flexion helped counteract the constant tugging of her spine into extension. Dawn was very active, so I gave her a standing exercise to work on (Wall Slides, page 80). I also explained how to do this exercise while sitting by flattening her lower spine against the back of a chair. Although she preferred sleeping

During the second and third trimester, lying down on your back (supine) can restrict blood flow to the fetus by pressing on a major blood vessel, the vena cava. **Consult your physician** when considering exercising or resting on your back.

on her side, I explained that she could also lie down on her back while keeping her knees bent, which helped push her lower back flat against the floor. This reduced the extreme lordotic curve of her lower spine. Be sure to run this recommendation by your physician though because you shouldn't spend too much time on your back later in pregnancy.

She called me two days later and said her sciatic pain was gone, but she was still having trouble with back pain on her walks.

"Let me guess," I said. "It hurts going downhill but feels better going uphill."

"Yes!" she said. "How did you know that?"

Now that you understand the mechanics of the spine, you might be able to guess how I deduced that she would feel better walking uphill. If you remember, the key to preventing back pain during pregnancy is to flex the lumbar spine, countering the excessive extension it adopts and reducing the lordotic curve, especially during the final trimester. When walking downhill, we must extend backwards to offset the forward momentum and slope of the hill. This causes back pain in pregnant women because they're already coping with too much extension. When walking uphill, we must flex forward to accommodate the slope. Flexing forward reduces back pain in pregnant women. Therefore walking uphill would result in less back pain than walking downhill. Elementary, my dear Watson!

> **Pregnancy belts,** designed to carry the weight of the fetus, work because they **relieve extension stress to the spine**. Unloading the weight of the fetus means the pelvis doesn't anteriorly tilt as readily. This reduces stress to the **SI joint, back, and pelvis**.

TESTING 1, 2, 3...

Now it's time to put all this information to the test and confirm that excessive extension is really what's hurting your back or contributing to sciatic pain. Get out a piece of paper and a pencil, and write down your answers to the following questions. You'll notice these tests require you to perform routine daily motions. Bring your attention to these motions to see which ones hurt you and which ones help you. Depending on where you are in your pregnancy, some of the tasks may be difficult for you. Skip these, please. The title of the book is *Fixing You,* not *Breaking You!*

Testing for Flexion & Extension Problems

1. Stand in a normal position. Do you have back pain?
Yes / No

2. Bend down and reach toward your toes. Does your back feel better or worse when you are flexed forward?
Better / Worse

3. Return to standing. Does your pain increase or decrease while returning to an upright position?
Increase / Decrease

4. Lean against a wall, flattening your lower back against it. You may have to bend your knees or walk your feet away from the

wall to flatten your lower back without straining. Does your pain increase or decrease when your lower back is flattened against the wall?

Increase / Decrease

5.   Sit in a chair. Press your lower back into the back of the chair. Does your pain increase or decrease?

Increase / Decrease

6.   Lie on your back (supine) on a firm surface, such as the floor. Let your body relax. Extend your legs so they rest on the floor with your knees straight. Stay there for approximately one minute. Walk your feet back to your rear, bending your knees, and stop at a comfortable position. Stay there for approximately one minute. Which position is more comfortable? If there is no difference, pull your knees up to your chest and hold them there for one minute, then assess.

Legs extended / Legs flexed (knees bent)

People with extension problems typically give the following answers:

1.   Yes
2.   Better
3.   Increase
4.   Decrease
5.   Decrease
6.   Legs flexed (knees bent)

As I said before, almost all back pain during pregnancy is due to excessive spinal extension, and hopefully you have a set of clear responses that confirms this (if not please read *Fixing You: Back Pain* to resolve your flexion problem). This is where many people have "Aha!" moments and understand why doing X hurts them, but doing Y is fine. Okay, so now that you understand a major contributor to your back pain, what can you do about it? In general, you need to allow your spine to relax in a flatter position by introducing more flexion as often as you can to unload the extension stress. The exercises in Section 3: Corrective Exercises will help you accomplish this.

Rotation Problems

Remember those muscles in the front of the pelvis that can tighten up and pull it forward into an anterior pelvic tilt? Well, as luck would have it, they don't always become tight symmetrically. Sometimes the muscles on one side of the pelvis become tighter than those on the other side. This creates a rotated pelvis—which then, of course, contributes to a rotated spine. Remember, the pelvis is the keystone to spinal function. Just how does this happen, you might ask? Rotation problems are often due to habits in how we stand, sit, or walk.

Shifting your weight to one leg while you're standing is a classic example of a habit that contributes to pelvic rotation. During a typical weight shift, the majority of your weight is transferred to one leg—let's say the left, for example; then your left knee straightens to accept the weight. Straightening your knee means your muscles don't need to work as hard. Instead, your knee and hip joints carry the load with minimal muscular effort. This is a nice way to give those aching leg muscles a rest, but it comes at a price. In this same example, the right knee usually bends and rotates inward slightly. When this happens often enough, the muscles controlling the bending and inward rotation of the right leg become tighter than those on the left. Can you guess which muscles? You've got it—the TFL, quadriceps, and (sometimes) sartorius muscles. When the right leg eventually straightens up, those same muscles pull the right side of the pelvis forward, which creates a rotated pelvis (Figure 2.9, page 42).

When the pelvis is rotated, often the spine will become side-bent (and therefore rotated), similar to what's happening in Figure 2.9. If this is a habitual posture, then your body will eventually develop a rotation problem (see Figures 2.10 and 2.11, page 43).

The woman on the next page has a side-bent and rotated spine. This occurred due to poor habits and asymmetrical tightness of the muscles at the front of her pelvis.

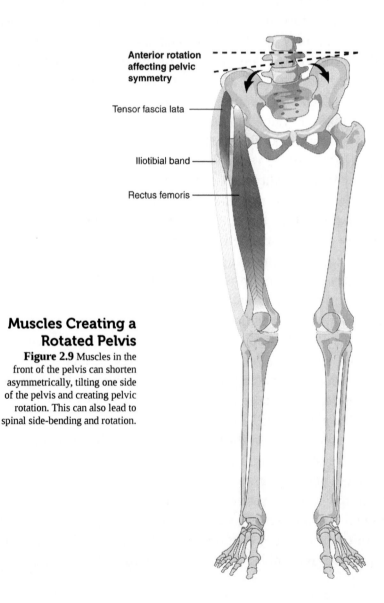

Anterior rotation affecting pelvic symmetry

Tensor fascia lata

Iliotibial band

Rectus femoris

Muscles Creating a Rotated Pelvis

Figure 2.9 Muscles in the front of the pelvis can shorten asymmetrically, tilting one side of the pelvis and creating pelvic rotation. This can also lead to spinal side-bending and rotation.

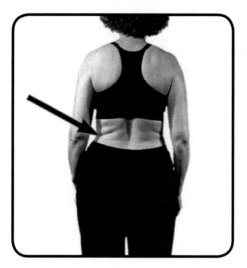

Side-Bending Posture

Figure 2.10 This woman's spine is habitually side-bent to the left. There is a larger crease on her left side than on her right (see arrow). Her spine is therefore rotated to the right. Note the paraspinal muscles along the right side of her spine are thicker than those on the left.

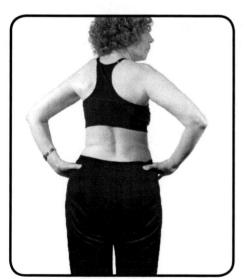

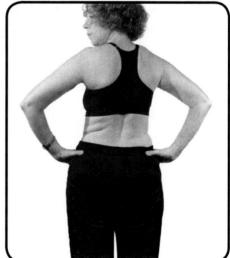

Right Rotation   Left Rotation

Spinal Rotation

Figure 2.11 This woman has limited left rotation and greater right spinal rotation. This is consistent with her permanent left side-bent position. Note the increased head rotation to the left during left rotation to "assist" her deficient left trunk rotation.

Ask yourself the following questions to help you zero in on habits that might contribute to rotation issues:

• **While watching TV,** do you typically sit on one side of the TV so that you must rotate to watch it? Do you typically sit with your legs rotated underneath you in a particular direction?

• **During your morning routine,** do you stand or sit with your trunk rotated or bear weight asymmetrically when you get your morning coffee, brush your teeth, or read the newspaper?

• **Do you play sports** that require stronger or more frequent rotation to one side than the other?

• **Do you sleep** on one side more than the other?

• **While driving,** do you tend to have one hand on the steering wheel? Are your hips equally bearing your weight?

• **While standing,** is one hip more forward than the other? Do you stand with one knee bent and the other straight? Do you bear more weight on one leg than the other?

• **While exercising,** do you run, elliptical, or bike with your trunk rotated? Are both legs symmetrically bearing your weight?

• **At the office,** is your office chair aligned with your desk? Is the desk organized so that you use both halves equally? Do you frequently turn to the same side to answer the phone? Check the time? Read a chart? Reach into files?

Now that you have an idea of what a side-bent or rotated spine looks like, let's get out a piece of paper and pencil to see whether your spine is rotated or not. You'll need someone's help to figure this out. I recommend a physical therapist, but I think the instructions are clear enough to have a friend help you out with this one. Again, please don't injure yourself to perform a test. You'll have a good idea of whether you are rotated or not even after skipping a couple tests.

Testing for Rotation Problems

1. Feel the paraspinal muscles (those that lie vertically on either side of the lumbar spine). Is one side smaller or thinner than the other?

Yes / No
If so, which side? Right / Left

2. Place your hands on your pelvis and hold your pelvis steady while rotating your upper body to the right. Then rotate it to the left. Which direction rotates more or has less pain?

Right / Left / Both are the same

3. Stand with hands at your sides. Now side-bend to the right, sliding your hand down your leg. Return to standing and side-bend to the left. Which side felt smoother, more natural, or had less pain?

Right / Left / Both are the same

4. Lie down on your right side for one minute. Then, lie down on your left side for one minute. Is it more painful or less comfortable to lie on one side than the other?

Right / Left / No difference

Answers to these questions are fairly obvious. If the majority of the answers indicate asymmetry, then chances are you have a rotation problem. The good news is that, in most cases, a rotated spine exacerbates back pain from either extension or flexion problems rather than being the primary issue. So focusing on correcting your extension issues will go a long way toward eliminating your pain. If it still persists, then you can also work on eliminating the rotation issues. Don't panic, though. Life is about asymmetry. You just need to learn to be a little less asymmetrical than you have been. You don't need to be perfect, just better than you are right now.

I usually begin by picking the most pervasive habit creating rotation, such as sitting while slightly rotated. Begin centering yourself, and eliminate uneven weight-bearing or weight-shifting habits. When watching TV, face it straight on. At work, put the items you use most in the center of your desk or distribute them equally to both sides. These changes will go a long way toward correcting your rotation problem.

You should also figure out whether your pelvis is rotated too. Remember, it may be the reason your spine is rotated in the first place. The two easy tests that follow will help you to do this. Again, I recommend a physical therapist perform these for you. However, if one is not available, I've tried to describe the process as simply as possible. These instructions can also be found as videos on my website, **www.FixingYou.net**, by typing in the code at the back of this book.

Testing for Pelvic Problems
1.   Standing on a level surface, have a friend or physical therapist kneel down with both hands on the tops of your pelvic bones (**iliac crests**) as in the picture below (Figure 2.12). Determine whether one side is higher than the other. Differences of 1/4 inch or greater can indicate pelvic rotation.

Checking
Iliac Crest Height
Figure 2.12 Kneel down so that your eyes are level with the waist to assess iliac crest height.

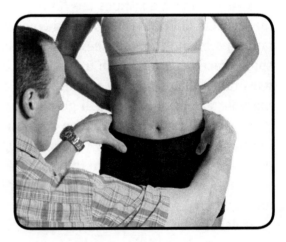

2. Next, slide your thumbs down and forward until you find a prominent ridge on the front of the pelvis. These are the **anterior superior iliac spines (ASISs)**. Keep sliding your thumbs over the ASISs until they just drop off into a more fleshy part of the hip. Stop when you reach these edges of the ASISs and assess the height difference. Usually (but not always) if one iliac crest is high, then the opposite ASIS will be low. Again, keep your eyes at the level of the pelvis to get a good look, as in Figure 2.13.

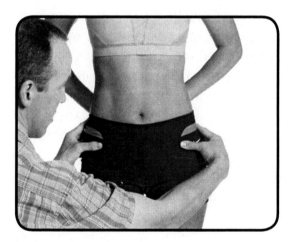

Checking ASIS Height

Figure 2.13 Use your thumbs when checking for differences in ASIS height.

If both tests indicate level landmarks, don't assume your pelvis is perfect—especially if you found that you have an extension problem. It's likely that both sides are equally tilted forward and are contributing to excessive extension in the lumbar spine. This may be due to tightness in the TFL and quadriceps muscles. You can determine if this is the issue and correct it by performing the TFL & Quadriceps Stretch (page 72) in Section 3: Corrective Exercises. If these muscles aren't tight, then your spine is probably biased toward an excessive lordotic curve, and you should focus on abdominal strengthening together with correcting poor habits, like locking your knees when you stand, that feed this movement dysfunction.

LOOKING CLOSELY AT THE SI JOINT

Okay, since we're talking about the pelvis, where does SI joint pain come in? SI joint pain or dysfunction is a common diagnosis, but what to do about it seems to puzzle a lot of people. You already have a greater understanding of what's at the root of this issue after reading to this point. Knowing that the pelvis is subject to unequal forces acting on it by the TFL and quadriceps muscles, and that the pelvic bones are more mobile than usual during pregnancy, it's not too far a stretch to imagine that this may play out at the SI joint. One ilia is being pulled forward more than the other by these muscles, which causes pain in the back of the pelvis. And if you understand that, then you probably can already guess how to fix it. You bet—the TFL & Quadriceps Stretch, for starters. The other part of the puzzle is identifying which habits contribute to this asymmetrical pulling. Seems pretty simple, right?

Well, not so fast. During the latter months of pregnancy, the ligaments holding the three bones of the pelvis together often become lax due to the hormone relaxin. This allows the ligaments to become ever-so-slightly looser and can cause pelvic pain that is sometimes diagnosed as SI joint pain. This can happen on one or both sides. The TFL & Quadriceps Stretch will almost always eliminate this stress and reduce pain. However, in those cases where the pelvic bones have become particularly loose, a belt tightened around the hip joints can help reduce pain as well. The belt essentially compresses the SI joint, holding it together again and eliminating pain.

> In the last trimester of pregnancy, it's a good idea to **reduce asymmetrical strengthening exercises**, such as lunging, to avoid stressing the SI joint area or contributing to pelvic or spinal rotation.

Client Connection: Helping Heather's Hips

Heather, a pregnant friend of mine, had invited us over for a party. While there, she mentioned she had constant pelvic pain now that she was in her third trimester. She described it as deep, aching, and sometimes sharp. I could see it was bothering her and asked if I could take a look. I knelt down beside her and squeezed her hips together.

"Oh my god! That feels so good!" she said. "It totally takes my pain away. Can you just stay there for the evening?"

I didn't think her husband would have appreciated that, so I asked her to get his belt. I cinched it around her hips, and voilà! No pain.

In the third trimester, the pelvis becomes wider while ligaments begin to relax in preparation for the baby's impending birth. This, together with the baby's weight, separates and strains the pelvic joints. I merely relieved the strain by compressing the bones together and holding them in position with a belt. You can use an ordinary belt or purchase a special belt online at rehabilitation or pregnancy websites.

By the way, this also worked for her ankle pain, which she had asked me about earlier (now that I think about it, she really owes me a favor!). She described her ankles as being achy, especially at the end of the day. As she was lying on her couch, I squeezed her ankle bones together. Her pain immediately went away. Ankles are similar to the pelvis; two bones compose either side and flank a third bone. Because her ligaments had relaxed as a result of her hormones and her weight had increased, the ankle bones had partially separated, which caused pain. I recommended she go to the local drugstore and get a pair of ankle braces to stabilize the joints.

Now are you getting the idea about how your back and pelvis work? Let's recap here to make sure we're all on the same page. The pelvis is the keystone to a healthy spine. During pregnancy, the pelvis often tips forward into an anterior pelvic tilt. This makes the spine arch back to offset the new pelvic position. This is so gradual, you won't even notice it—until you have pain.

When the pelvis tips forward, the muscles in front of the pelvis can become tight, locking it in this position. This tilt creates an excessive lordotic curve. Consequently, the spine remains in extension even when bending forward. This continual lumbar extension eventually causes pain. This is called an extension problem. Depending on the person, one side of the muscles in the front of the pelvis can become tighter than the other side, creating a rotated pelvis. This can create a rotated spine. That's it in a nutshell so far. Let's move on to the next piece of the puzzle, your abdominal muscles.

LOOKING CLOSELY AT THE ABDOMINAL MUSCLES

The abdominal muscles prove to be a difficult area to tackle during and after pregnancy. Hopefully, the following information will help you regain good function and tone or at least help you understand why you're not there yet.

The abdominals consist of four muscles: the **rectus abdominus**, **internal** and **external obliques**, and **transversus abdominus**. The rectus abdominus starts at the front of the ribcage where the ribs meet and inserts onto the pubic bones of the pelvis. The obliques (internal and external) crisscross and run from the more lateral part of the ribcage and insert onto the top and front of the ilia. The transversus abdominus wraps around the gut starting at the spine, then grabs the lower ribs and inserts into the central vertical line of the abdominal muscles (Figure 2.14).

> The integrity of the **linea alba** can be compromised as a result of pregnancy, which affects the abdominal muscles' ability to **stabilize the spine**.

This tendinous central line is called the **linea alba**. It runs from the pelvis up to the sternum, and all the abdominals attach into it. When the pelvis is tilted forward in an anterior pelvic tilt, the abdominal muscles become lengthened. This compromises their ability to stabilize the spine. There are varying degrees of anterior pelvic tilt, and it differs from person to person. Correcting anterior pelvic tilt is necessary to allow the abdominals to stabilize the spine. This is especially true for people who have an extension or rotation problem.

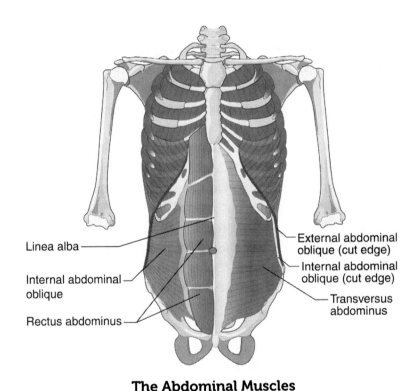

The Abdominal Muscles

Figure 2.14 The abdominals consist of four muscles, all of which insert into the linea alba.

During pregnancy, these abdominal muscles also become more stretched out because of the fetus's increasing size. They lose some of the force they were able to generate prior to pregnancy. Think of a rubber band that has been stretched for a while and then released. It doesn't just snap back on its own. The good news is that, unlike a rubber band, your abdominal muscles can regain their strength and tension again with some effort on your part. Specific training will be required (Heel Slides and Knee Wobbles, pages 82 and 84), but the payoff will be preventing back pain down the road—as well as slimming your tummy faster.

Your abdominal muscles may also have separated during your pregnancy, causing a condition after pregnancy known as **diastasis recti**. This happens along the linea alba, which divides the abdominals into left and right halves. As I mentioned, all the abdominal muscles attach here. Their ability to stabilize the spine is compromised when the linea alba is separated too far. Yes, this thin tendinous line can actually separate, creating a gap. The bigger the gap, the less tension and therefore stabilization will be generated by the abdominal muscles. Compound this with increased lordosis and an anterior pelvic tilt, and you've got a recipe for back pain. Amazingly, most insurance companies do not see this separation as a necessary repair but instead have relegated it to plastic surgery. Let's perform a little test to see if you have a separation and how big it is. This test should be performed a couple weeks or so after your baby is born. Doing it during pregnancy will not only be difficult but will also give a false result.

Diastasis Recti Test

To test whether you have a significant separation, lie down on your back with your knees bent. Place your fingers over the center of your abdomen. Nod your chin to your chest and lift your shoulders just a little while contracting your abdominal muscles (you're essentially performing an abdominal crunch). Feel the distance between the left and right halves of the abdominal muscles with your fingers, starting at the top and moving down the length toward your pubic bones (Figure 2.15). It will be separated less or more depending where you are feeling along this line, so take your time to assess its whole length. Typically, the widest separation will be close to the belly button.

Is there a gap running down the middle of your stomach equal to or less than two fingers' width? If so, then you have a mild separation that will probably resolve with correct conditioning. Current wisdom states that a linea alba separation equal to or less than two finger widths is not a significant separation. My belief is that if you have back pain and are unable to generate enough abdominal tension to stabilize it, even half a finger's width is too much.

A pronounced separation wider than two and a half fingers requires more attention. If you see a small bulge protruding, this may be a herniation; you should contact your physician. In this circumstance, exercise caution when lifting, sitting up, and performing rotating activities.

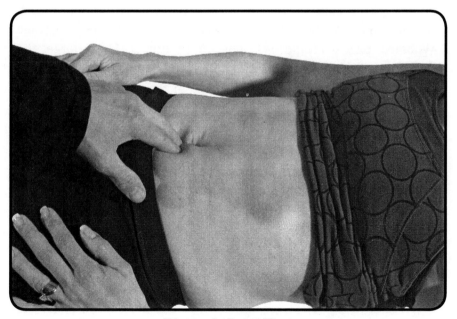

Diastasis Recti Test

Figure 2.15 A separation greater than two fingers' width can potentially compromise the integrity of core spine-stabilizing muscles. This woman had surgery to pull her abdominal muscles back together again. Even after surgery, however, they maintain a separation of two fingers' width.

A video clip of this test can be found at **www.FixingYou.net**. Just enter the code found at the back of this book to access all the assessment and rehabilitative exercises in this book.

You will notice the woman in the Figure 2.15 has excellent abdominal muscle tone. However, this tone is limited to the rectus abdominus muscles—the ones that form the six-pack ridges of the stomach. Her deeper, spinal-stabilizing muscles were actually very weak. In fact, she had a difficult time contracting them at all. Her training program included lots of crunches, which developed her six-pack look but did relatively little to develop her deeper spinal-stabilizing abdominal muscles. She was very active and came to me with nagging back pain. We identified the biomechanical issues contributing to her back pain, gave her corrective exercises, and began an appropriate tummy-strengthening program to stabilize her spine.

With a significant abdominal muscle separation, crunches and sit-ups are not appropriate and may even make the problem worse. Instead, perform the abdominal exercises (Heel Slides and Knee Wobbles, pages 82 and 84) listed in Section 3. These target the deeper stabilizing muscles, which need to become stronger to pull in the abdominal contents and reduce bulging of the abdomen. It will initially be difficult to get the muscles to contract due to their stretched condition. Keep trying! They will eventually respond. Even if you don't have a separation, begin with these exercises to stabilize any increase in lumbar lordosis due to the pregnancy. Jumping in to other exercises without

Diastasis Recti

If a separation greater than two and a half fingers' width is noted, caution should be exercised when:

1. **performing certain activities** that involve extending the spine, such as lying over an exercise ball or the yoga position Upward-Facing Dog;

2. **performing abdominal exercises** such as crunches that overly recruit (and possibly further separate) the rectus abdominus;

3. **coughing,** which will also protrude the rectus abdominus;

4. **lifting** heavy objects.

first activating the deeper stabilizing muscles could lead to injury.

Current wisdom frowns upon physically closing a separation with your hands by pushing the abdomi-

Brisk, forceful exhaling will help activate deeper core muscles needed for spinal stabilization.

nals together. Instead, most people recommend training the abdominals to do this. But how can the abdominal muscles close the gap if they're too separated to generate adequate force? Therefore, I allow my clients to hold the two halves of their abdominals together while they perform strengthening exercises if the muscles are unable to achieve this on their own.

The take-home message from this is that pregnancy not only stretches the abdominal muscles but can also make it difficult to regain their strength due to the pelvis stuck in an anterior pelvic tilt or separation of the linea alba. Having one or both of these conditions means you must be extra vigilant about what you are doing in terms of exercise and daily activities. Therefore, it would help if you began the abdominal strengthening exercises mentioned here early in your pregnancy to gain a sense of how your muscles should perform and keep them as toned as possible throughout your pregnancy.

LOOKING CLOSELY AT MOVEMENT

Okay, now that we've seen how pregnancy can affect your spine, pelvis, and abdominals, let's put it all together to see what happens when you move. If you remember, I mentioned the pelvis is the keystone to spine function. When you walk, sit, lie down, lift, or do any other activity, the spine and pelvis must work together to allow pain-free movement.

You've seen how pregnancy can create a pelvis that is anteriorly tilted, which in turn alters the lordotic curve of the spine as well as abdominal function. Now let's see how this plays out when you do one of the most commonly repeated activities during the day—bending down to pick something up.

Ideally, your pelvis should flex forward with your spine as you bend forward. The timing of this pelvic flexion is very important. Think of the pelvis as a guide for the spine; when you bend forward, both your spine and pelvis move together to prevent excessive stress from irritating the spine (Figure 2.16).

When women have extension problems, the pelvis typically flexes too soon or too much and the spine remains in extension

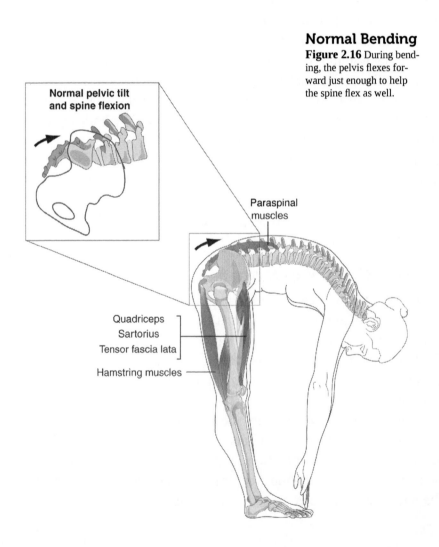

Normal Bending

Figure 2.16 During bending, the pelvis flexes forward just enough to help the spine flex as well.

Normal pelvic tilt and spine flexion

Paraspinal muscles

Quadriceps
Sartorius
Tensor fascia lata
Hamstring muscles

(Figure 2.17). Part of the reason this happens is the hamstring muscles in the back of the legs become too long, which allows the pelvis to tilt forward excessively. As a result, the muscles along the spine controlling spinal extension, the paraspinal muscles, become short or tight (Figure 2.18, page 58). The further you are into your pregnancy, the harder it will be to change this dynamic. However, there are plenty of things to do to relieve pain and make

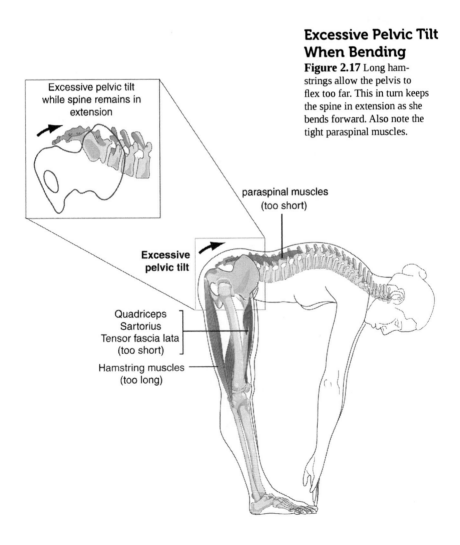

Excessive Pelvic Tilt When Bending

Figure 2.17 Long hamstrings allow the pelvis to flex too far. This in turn keeps the spine in extension as she bends forward. Also note the tight paraspinal muscles.

Excessive pelvic tilt while spine remains in extension

paraspinal muscles (too short)

Excessive pelvic tilt

Quadriceps
Sartorius
Tensor fascia lata
(too short)

Hamstring muscles
(too long)

changes where you can. We'll cover these shortly.

When you bent over to touch the floor while testing yourself for extension problems, you probably felt a nice stretch in your lower back at the bottom of that bending movement. That's because your pelvis had flexed forward as far as it could, so the spine was finally able to flex, which stretched the paraspinal muscles. These muscles get achy when they're overworked all day, as is the case when the spine is overly extended.

When returning to a standing position from bending over, the spine typically extends first, contracting those same paraspinal muscles. This is where major back pain starts because the spine is extending, exerting tremendous force, at the most mobile vertebrae. Once again, this usually occurs at the lumbosacral junction. You may have noticed this pattern during the previous testing.

The abdominals won't be of much help to stabilize the spine because they are most likely too stretched out. So the spine is on its own, absorbing the stress at a hypermobile segment again and again.

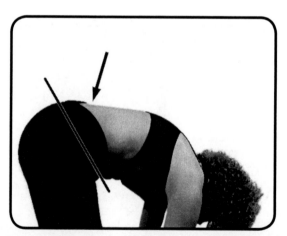

Excessive Pelvic Flexion During Bending

Figure 2.18 This woman does not allow her spine to bend while flexing forward, creating excessive stress at her most mobile vertebrae. Note the straight line indicating the pelvic flexion due, in part, to her extreme hamstring length.

How can we fix this pattern? You're taking the first step right now by becoming familiar with this information. Now you must apply it. Every little thing you can do will help. Let's begin by bending your knees and allowing the spine

If you have an extension problem, rest against the back of a chair when sitting. This allows the lumbar spine to flatten, relieving pain.

to bend (flex) sooner than normal when bending forward. This allows your pelvis to flex forward more slowly and your paraspinal muscles to stretch sooner during the movement. When returning upright from bending forward, walk your hands up your thighs to help unload the weight of your upper body and maintain a flexed spine longer. As you return to a standing position, visualize the top of your pelvis tipping backward (into a posterior pelvic tilt). To help visualize this, imagine that you have a tail, and "tuck it" between your legs. If you imitate this motion, your rear end will tuck underneath you into a posterior pelvic tilt. This helps flatten the spine. You can also "hollow out" your stomach by drawing your belly button in toward your spine. By doing this, your spine flexes and remains in flexion as you stand upright, which allows your vertebrae to stack up on one another rather than hinge at just one level of the spine. This will allow your paraspinal muscles to remain lengthened and distribute stress equally to all the lumbar vertebrae, rather than just the most mobile ones. These two changes should have considerable effect on your back pain. I demonstrate this in the video clips on my website, **www.FixingYou.net**, which you can access by typing in the code at the back of this book.

Let's recap what we've learned. We've covered just about everything you need to know about the sources of your pain and how to fix them. You now understand why your back is more inclined to experience pain as your pregnancy progresses. The increased curvature of the lumbar spine causes stress to the tissues surrounding the most mobile vertebrae, usually at the lumbosacral junction. This also affects how you bend forward and straighten back up. You've learned that your back pain will be reduced by flexing your spine. Flexing your spine while bending forward and straightening up will have a dramatic effect on your pain. You've also learned how all these factors in combination with a wider pelvis contribute to sciatic pain, and how to alleviate stress to these nerve roots during the day and while sleeping.

The pelvis, the keystone of spinal mechanics, often becomes anteriorly tilted as your pregnancy progresses. This tilt becomes more or less permanent because the muscles in the front of your pelvis shorten to accommodate the tilt; if they're not stretched later after the baby is born, they will continue to maintain the anterior pelvic tilt. In terms of movement, this anterior tilt keeps your spine in excessive extension when you bend over and stand up. This creates stress, and therefore pain, at the most mobile vertebrae. Slightly unlock your knees to help prevent your pelvis from flexing forward too soon and allow your spine to remain in some flexion—which reduces pain.

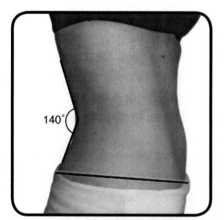 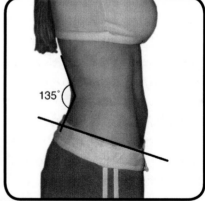

Residual Pelvic Tilt and Lordosis

Figure 2.19 Notice the neutral pelvis in the first picture, taken early in this woman's pregnancy. The second picture was taken nine months after her baby was born. Note the anterior pelvic tilt and increased lumbar lordosis.

Even if you've stayed in great shape before, during, and after your pregnancy, the dynamics of your spine and pelvis may have been considerably altered without your awareness. For many women, these dynamics don't just return to normal on their own (Figure 2.19). The woman in these pictures is young and obviously fit but unaware of the changes her body has undergone during and after pregnancy. Resuming an exercise program without first understanding if these changes have remained in place will, in most cases, merely emphasize the changes and possibly make them worse.

The exercises in Section 3 are designed to correct these changes and help you restore your body to its pre-pregnancy shape. Hopefully, you'll be even better than before!

Helpful Tips for Getting Through the Day

As your pregnancy develops, more stress will be placed on lax joints. It's important you find as many ways as you can to rest these joints throughout the day. To help relieve pain from extension problems, periodically sit down and flatten your spine against the back of a chair to remove excessive extension stress. Performing a Wall Slide (page 80) can also help if you are on your feet. At every opportunity, try to flatten your lumbar spine. Activate your deeper stabilizing abdominal muscles by drawing your belly button in toward your spine. You'll notice your spine likes to arch quite a bit while driving. Make it a habit to check and correct this habit at every stoplight. The All-Fours Rocking Stretch and Forward Bend Stretch are two easy exercises to periodically work into your routine to stave off pain. Simply holding your tummy with your hands will also decrease the stress pulling your spine into extension.

Women with rotation problems typically bear more weight on one leg than the other. When standing or sitting, pay attention to your posture and become more symmetrical. Another common habit is leaning to one side of your workstation while resting on an elbow. This creates side-bending and therefore rotation.

GET A GOOD NIGHT'S SLEEP

Sleeping habits are major contributors to back pain. Often, the TFL and quadriceps muscles pull the pelvis into an anterior pelvic tilt, which creates excessive lumbar lordosis (Figure 2.20). Put pillows under your knees to help relieve the pelvic tilt that causes your spine to arch. When sleeping on your side, pull your knees up to your chest to help reduce the excessive spinal extension and

Lumbar Lordosis When Lying Down

Figure 2.20 When lying on your back, tight pelvic mucles help create excessive lumbar lordosis and back pain.

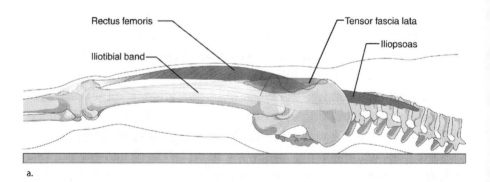

Rectus femoris

Tensor fascia lata

Iliopsoas

Iliotibial band

a.

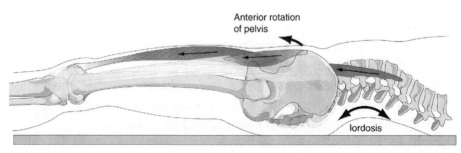

Anterior rotation of pelvis

lordosis

b.

relieve pain. Putting pillows between your knees will help alleviate stress to hip muscles that can become irritated later. This also helps eliminate sciatic pain. Perform the All-Fours Rocking Stretch or TFL & Quadriceps Stretch

> If you believe your pain has more to do with your hips or pelvis, please read **Fixing You: Hip & Knee Pain.**

(pages 75 and 72) before going to bed to help reduce pain while you sleep.

As your pregnancy progresses, your pelvis becomes wider in anticipation of the baby's birth. Sleeping on your side with wider hips subjects your spine to more side-bending and, therefore, rotation (Figure 2.21). This side-bending coupled with rotation can often impinge nerve roots that exit the spine, which compose the sciatic nerve. In Dawn's case, her spine was already rotated to one direction—the right. Therefore, she felt pain when she rotated to the left.

Typically, the spine will resist rotation at the least mobile vertebrae and instead side-bend and rotate at the most mobile segment(s). Lying on the other side doesn't cause pain because

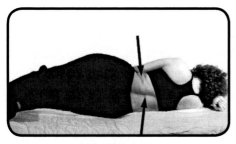
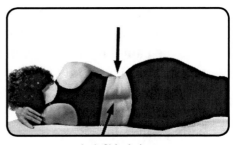

Right Side-Lying   **Left Side-Lying**

Sleeping Positions

Figure 2.21 Lying on your side introduces side-bending and therefore spinal rotation to the opposite direction. Notice this woman is able to side-bend more when lying on her right side (evidenced by more wrinkles in her side) than her left. The muscles along the spine are more relaxed because this position favors her right-rotated spine. The muscles along the spine in the left side-lying picture are more stressed than those in the picture on the right because her spine is being forced to side-bend and rotate in a direction it is not accustomed to (notice the lack of creases on her waist). She has increased pain lying on this side.

the spine's rotation favors that direction (see Figure 2.21, page 63). A towel placed under your waist will diminish side-bending of the spine and therefore rotation and **impingement** of the nerve roots. When rolling over to the other side, the towel will again serve to neutralize the spine's side-bending and rotation. This can also reduce irritation of the sciatic nerve.

"THROWING YOUR BACK OUT": CORRECTIVE MEASURES FOR ACUTE INJURY

I often hear clients say they've "thrown out" their backs. This phrase is applied to sudden, crippling pain caused by any number of factors that often relate to vertebrae that are moving too much. In my experience, manipulation or mobilization of the spine only adds to the problem. Stabilization is what's needed.

Lie on your back with knees bent and your lower legs up on a chair or stool. This position unloads the disks between the vertebrae and the tissues interacting with them, such as certain hip flexor muscles. Get into this position and just try to relax. Ice is often helpful to reduce the pain.

Those with extension problems will benefit from letting their backs relax into the floor, supporting the lower spine or flattening it out a bit. Those with rotation problems may find that a folded towel under one hip or under one side of their lower backs helps ease the pain. Find the position that works best for you and maintain it. The first priority is to let the irritated nerves calm down.

As the pain subsides and while in ideal alignment, gently practice stabilizing your back by firing your abdominals. Forceful exhaling will help activate these muscles.

Then you can move into a sitting position in which your back is supported similarly to your position on the floor. Rest and allow the nerves to calm down. Your muscles' ability to adequately stabilize your spine is compromised under conditions of severe pain because pain inhibits muscle function. Therefore a little help is needed. Place your hands below your belly, cupping the baby, and lift slightly. This will remove much of the stress that's adding to your problem. Special slings are available to purchase online that will help unload the weight of the baby, which will remove the extension stress on your spine.

Eventually, try standing with your back up against the wall for support in the same manner as it was supported while sitting. Stabilize your spine. Gradually walk away from the wall with your spine stabilized to protect it. You may not get any further than one step before you feel the need to lean against the wall again. That's okay. Return to the wall and relax your back again. Continue attempting to walk with your spine stabilized and in good alignment.

CONCLUSION

Most statistics say that back pain during pregnancy resolves on its own within about three months after giving birth. It's no wonder because the main protagonist is now lying in a crib! But not having back pain doesn't mean that all the issues that created it during your pregnancy have resolved. It just means they've resolved enough that you don't have back pain right now. As you've seen, your body doesn't necessarily bounce back on its own. You'll need to take specific steps to correct many of the changes that have occurred to your pelvis and spine.

Many women continue to have increased lordosis years after giving birth because they didn't retrain their spines to adopt their normal posture, or they didn't know to stretch the TFL and quadriceps muscles to restore normal pelvic position (Figure 2.19, page 60). Correcting both these issues will expedite abdominal strengthening by restoring the muscles' normal length and tension. Taking time to work on these issues now can prevent future back pain as well as help your tummy-toning program.

Especially with health care costs spiraling out of control, doesn't it make sense to take a little time now to make sure you won't have expensive, time-consuming, life-altering pain in the future? Back pain can cost insurance companies hundreds of thousands of dollars and can cost you quality time with family and friends, as well as out-of-pocket expenses for treatment.

I believe the changes to a mother's body are overlooked problems in postpartum care. A woman's body is altered by the experience of being pregnant, and specific attention is needed to restore it to its former shape. It is assumed the mother will just "bounce back" after the pregnancy. More attention is given to fixing a sprained ankle than to the physical changes a new mother has undergone after growing a baby for nine months. Take the time to understand how these issues have played out in your body. I hope this book will be a good start for your complete and healthy recovery!

3 | CORRECTIVE EXERCISES

I've been a few places like that where I've thought, "A BREAKTHROUGH *is possible here. This is the place for the* EXERCISES *that will bring me to* WHERE I WANT TO BE. *"*

—JOSEPH CAMPBELL

The following exercises are meant to develop strength and improve range of motion. Restoring range of motion and getting your body moving the way it should always helps healing and reduces pain. This is tricky, especially for those of you in your third trimester, so after you consult with your physician, you'll need to experiment a little to find the best solutions for you. If you find a particular exercise difficult, decide whether this is due to range-of-motion or strength issues, or because the exercise is awkward to perform, given your condition. Chances are, it is due to weakness or movement dysfunction. Take that as a cue that you need help in that area and therefore should practice it until you've mastered it. Good form is critical.

Resist the temptation to push too far too fast, and remember to **listen to your body**. If you feel pain, stop!

If you find an exercise that feels good, then do it as often as you can. Trust your body, it knows what it likes! In particular, the stretches should always feel good. It's a good idea to begin with stretching to identify the exercise(s) that will do the most good for you. During the first week or two, I typically begin with stretches such as the All-Fours Rocking Stretch, Forward Bend Stretch, or TFL & Quadriceps Stretch. These will really reduce your back pain.

Poor form or posture during strength training can promote back pain. Understand your poor habits and **counter them with good form.**

Stretching exercises are generally held for 30 to 60 seconds. Performing two to five repetitions is usually all that's needed to experience a positive effect. I typically ask my clients to commit to performing their stretches as often as possible (two to five times each day) during the first week or two to aggressively reduce their symptoms. In fact, the All-Fours Rocking Stretch is so effective, I ask my clients to perform this every time they experience pain. It should always feel good to perform the stretching exercises, so this really shouldn't be a hard sell. You should feel that your pain has decreased as a result. After the symptoms have abated, you can cut down on the frequency of stretching and find the ideal number of times needed to keep your pain at bay. I recommend doing them at least first thing in the morning and last thing before bed, as most people's back pain is aggravated during sleep.

After the stretching phase, begin strengthening. Add one exercise at a time to focus on getting it right and to test whether your pain is made worse by a particular exercise. If it is made worse, then either your technique is incorrect or it's not the right exercise for you. Pay attention to how you are performing the exercise. Read the instructions carefully and watch the video clips on the Fixing You website at **www.FixingYou.net**. Type in the code at the back of the book to access the free clips. Once you are successfully performing the exercise, then layer on the next. Each time you add a new strengthening exercise, don't change anything else about your program. This way, you'll be able to isolate which exercise may be causing pain.

> **If you are weight training,** you may find that you **must temporarily decrease the weight** you are using. It's okay—fixing your back is the **bigger picture.**

As you learned earlier, when your abdominals are stretched out by the baby, it will be harder to find and activate them. Be patient; it will come. Focus on keeping your spine flat, such as during the Heel Slides exercise, and you will automatically turn on those hard-to-find abdominal muscles.

Strengthening exercises generally require 5 to 10 repetitions for one to two sets or until fatigue or compensatory movements occur. Just a little bit of strengthening is needed to effect a positive change. As always, quality is more important than quantity. Strengthening exercises only need to be performed two to three times per day.

The exercises on the next page are the ones that I've found give most people almost immediate relief. Begin with these, focusing on range of motion. Once you have mastered them, progress to the strengthening exercises.

Finally, I'd like to emphasize again that you should consult your physician prior to beginning these exercises. There can be many causes of back and pelvic pain that are not musculoskeletal in nature, which should be addressed appropriately. Bring this book in to your physician to show him or her what you are planning.

Top 5 Exercises
for Back Pain During Pregnancy

❶ TFL & Quadriceps Stretch stretches key pelvic muscles that affect pelvic rotation and contribute to back pain. It also develops lower abdominal strength to resist pelvic rotation caused by tight thigh or pelvic muscles.

❷ All-Fours Rocking Stretch passively restores normal pelvic and spinal mechanics.

❸ Forward Bend Stretch stretches tight paraspinal muscles.

❹ Wall Slides develop core muscles for greater control of the lower spine while standing.

❺ Heel Slides develop core muscles for greater control of the lower spine.

TFL & QUADRICEPS STRETCH

This exercise stretches the muscles that attach to the front of the pelvis, which affect pelvic tilt and rotation and contribute to back, pelvic, and sciatic pain. The TFL & Quadriceps Stretch will also develop lower abdominal strength to resist pelvic rotation caused by tight thigh or pelvic muscles. During pregnancy, it is important to move slowly because the pelvic bones are looser and can rotate more easily. Be sure to stabilize your pelvis.

THE FIXING YOU METHOD—LEVEL 1

Lie on your back with both knees drawn to your chest. Hold your left knee with your left hand and arm. Depending on how far along you are, you may have to hold your knee to the outside of your chest because your belly is in the way. Place your right hand on the bony prominence (ASIS) of your right hip. Slowly lower your right leg to the floor with your knee bent. Then slide your right leg away from you, straightening your knee. Stop if your spine arches off the table or your pelvis rotates away from the table into your right hand. See if you can keep your back flat and your pelvis from rotating while your right leg rests on the floor. If necessary, pull your left knee into your chest with more force to help you. Note whether you feel a gentle stretch in your upper thigh close to your hip bone or in the mid or lower thigh muscles. Hold the stretch for 30–60 seconds, then switch legs. The goal here is to keep your back flat and not allow your pelvis to rotate forward while your right leg is fully stretched out. Adding a 5- to 10-pound weight to your right thigh (near your knee) may increase your stretch. Don't add weight until you can keep your back flat.

MODIFICATION FOR ROTATION PROBLEMS

You'll find that one side of your pelvis rotates more or sooner than the other side. Or you may find that it's more difficult to keep one side of your spine flat as compared to the other side. You must either stabilize against this rotation by using your lower abdominal muscles to stretch these muscles responsible for rotating the pelvis, or not allow that leg to fully extend until you are able to control your spine.

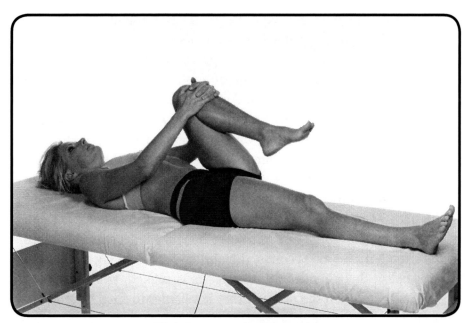

TFL & Quadriceps Stretch, Level 1

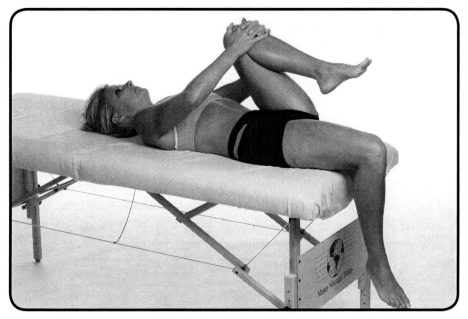

TFL & Quadriceps Stretch, Level 2

THE FIXING YOU METHOD—LEVEL 2

Level 2 of this exercise requires greater abdominal strength and control of the lumbar spine because it's a more aggressive stretch of the muscles in the front of the pelvis. Begin just as in Level 1, but lie down close to the edge of a table so that the leg you're lowering can drop below you. Again, let's say you're stretching the right side first. Begin with both knees to your chest (or slightly out to the side, depending on how big your belly is). Hold on to your left knee; keep your lower back flat on the table while you lower your right knee (bent to 90 degrees). Allow your leg to lower on its own; don't push it down. The goal is to keep your lumbar spine flat while your right leg lowers until your upper thigh can rest on the table with your knee bent at 90 degrees. Maintain the stretch for 30–60 seconds, then bring your right leg back up to your chest. Switch sides. If your pelvis is rotated, you'll find one side is tighter than the other or that it's harder to keep your lower back flat on the table.

COMMON ERRORS

- If you experience back pain while stretching, your abdominals aren't stabilizing your spine adequately, and your pelvis is rotating more than it should. Begin again and become more aware of when your spine starts to arch off the table. Stop there and let the tissues stretch. Remember, this is not a contest. You'll have plenty of time to stretch these muscles and develop awareness of your spine.

- If you stretch too aggressively, knee pain in the leg that's being lowered may result. Lower your leg only within a comfortable range of motion, or slide your leg out to the side and then lower it. Find a position where you can experience the stretch pain free. Your goal will then be to gradually work your way back in, so you can lower your leg straight down instead of out to the side.

ALL-FOURS ROCKING STRETCH

This exercise passively restores normal hip and spinal mechanics and feels great for the lower back when performed properly. Move only in a pain-free range of motion. Depending on how far along you are, this exercise may not be possible or advised by your physician. Consult your doctor first. You may find that he or she prefers the modified version.

THE FIXING YOU METHOD

Get on your hands and knees with your hands generally under your shoulders and knees under your hips. Depending on how far along you are, you may need to spread your knees out a bit to give your tummy clearance. In this position, you may find that your back sags down from the weight of your baby. Pull it up so it doesn't sag, and make sure your spine and pelvis are in neutral positions. Draw your belly button in toward your spine to help activate your abs and control your back. Rock back onto your feet while you keep your hands in place and maintain your neutral spine. Hold for 5 breaths. Repeat 5–10 times.

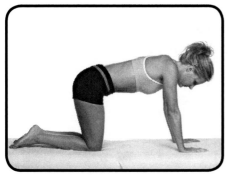

All-Fours Rocking Stretch,
start position

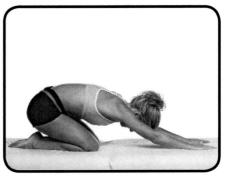

All-Fours Rocking Stretch,
end position

ALTERNATIVE ALL-FOURS ROCKING STRETCH

Sit in a chair and slide your arms forward over a low table; allow your shoulders to shrug up to your ears and your lower back to bend forward. Your knees should be separated to allow your belly to drop between them. You should feel a nice stretch in your lumbar spine as your back flexes. If the weight of the baby makes it too difficult for you to control your spine, you may want to place a pillow on a stool underneath you to gently rest your tummy on while you allow your spine to flex. Don't rest your entire weight on your tummy, but rather unload just a little of that extra weight to give you a chance to flex your spine.

MODIFICATION FOR ROTATION PROBLEMS

You'll find that one hip or one side of your spine is up higher than the other when you rock backward. For instance, your right hip may not come down toward your heel as far as your left hip, or your right paraspinal muscles may seem to bulge more than the left. In this case, scoot your right knee out to the side about 2–3 inches; keep your foot where it is. Rock back and feel that your hips or spine are more symmetrical. Find the right distance to scoot out your knee until you feel both your hips and/or spine are symmetrical. Repeat 5–10 times, then scoot your knee back in where you began and recheck. Continue repeating this sequence until you feel your spine or pelvis is symmetrical. It's often helpful to have someone watch you perform this exercise.

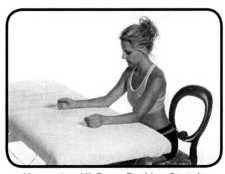

Alternative All-Fours Rocking Stretch,
start position

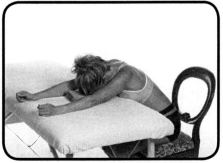

Alternative All-Fours Rocking Stretch,
end position

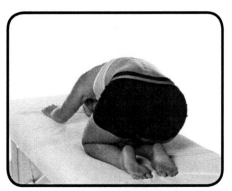

All-Fours Rocking Stretch,
rotation error

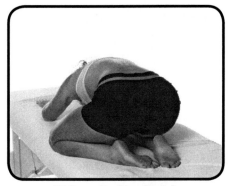

All-Fours Rocking Stretch,
rotation corrected

COMMON ERRORS

- When you rock back onto your heels, don't round your upper spine to help flatten your lower spine. All you need to do is flatten your lumbar spine a little more than you have been. Try to do this without rounding your upper spine.

- If you feel back pain during this exercise, determine at what point during the rocking back motion it begins to hurt. At that point, work extra hard to pull your belly up in order to flatten your spine. The other problem may be that your tummy is just too heavy for you to control, in which case this exercise isn't right for you.

- Be sure you line up with your knees under or slightly in front of your hip joints. When your knees are behind your hips, your back automatically increases its lordotic curve—which we don't want to happen.

- If your hips are painful during this exercise, scoot your knees out to the side about 2–3 inches away from your body, or only rock into a pain-free range of motion.

- If one hip doesn't go quite as far as the other when you rock back, then scoot that knee out to the side 2–3 inches to compensate for that rotation.

FORWARD BEND STRETCH

This exercise relieves strain to the lower spine by stretching tight back-extensor muscles that contribute to painful movement habits. These muscles get tighter and tighter as lumbar lordosis increases due to your growing baby.

THE FIXING YOU METHOD

Sit in a chair or on an exercise ball. Scoot to the edge and bend forward to stretch your lower back. Walk your hands down your legs to support your trunk. Stop if you feel any pain. Flex forward to the point where you can feel a pain-free stretch. You may have to scoot your legs out a little to accommodate your tummy. This should feel really good if you have extension problems. Many people experience pain when returning from the flexed position; if you feel pain, walk your hands up your legs to help return your trunk to an upright position. While coming back up, draw your belly button in toward your spine; maintain the lumbar flexion as long as possible. This maneuver is also called "hollowing out" your stomach. This exercise can also be done standing.

COMMON ERRORS

• If you have pain when you're coming back up, you need to flex your lumbar spine more; draw your belly button in toward your spine or use your hands to help push you back up or both.

• People with rotation problems should scoot the same knee out to the side as in the All-Fours Rocking exercise to prevent spinal rotation while stretching.

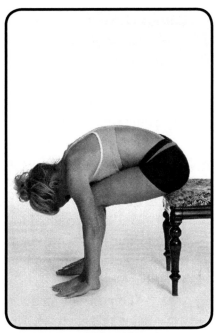

Forward Bend Stretch

WALL SLIDES

This is a functional exercise that teaches you to recruit lower abdominal muscles that support the spine while walking or standing. You need only do one repetition to correct your spine. Maintain that correction as you walk away from the wall.

THE FIXING YOU METHOD

Rest your back against the wall until it is flat or less extended by bending your knees and walking your feet away from the wall. Once your lower spine is flat, your back should feel much better. Now exhale while you slide your body up the wall and walk your feet toward the wall. As you slide up the wall, draw your belly button in toward your spine to prevent your back from arching again. Now step away from the wall while you maintain the contracted abs to stabilize your lumbar spine. See how long you can hold it. Don't forget to breathe! Whenever your back gets achy, you can return to this exercise, which will reset your lower abdominals to stabilize your spine.

COMMON ERRORS

• Some of you with heavy tummies will have trouble preventing your back from arching or getting it flat against the wall. All we care about is doing it well enough to eliminate your pain. Feel free to cup your belly with your hands to unload your baby's weight from your spine while you do this exercise.

• Try not to round your upper body in order to flatten your lower back against the wall. That just develops unnatural biomechanics and can lead to other problems. Remember, your spine doesn't need to be perfectly flat, just flexed enough to eliminate your pain.

• You'll be tempted to flatten your lumbar spine flat by pushing into the wall with your legs. This defeats the purpose. We're trying to develop your abdominal strength to hold your spine in a better position.

• Many of you might allow one of your knees to collapse in while doing this exercise. This promotes pelvic rotation, so please be aware of this and don't let it happen.

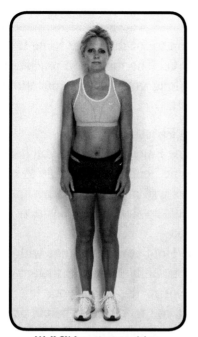 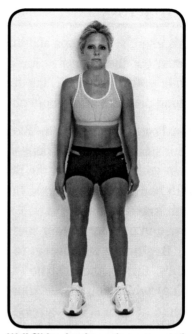

Wall Slides, start position   Wall Slides, lumbar spine supported

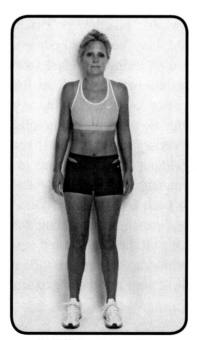

Wall Slides, end position

HEEL SLIDES

This exercise develops abdominal control of the lower spine to help flatten out the excessive lordotic curve. The more you practice this while you're pregnant, the further along you'll be in your tummy-toning program after your baby is born.

THE FIXING YOU METHOD—EXTENSION PROBLEMS

Your start position will depend on how much hip flexion you need to keep your spine flat on the floor. Some people will be able to begin with both feet on the floor, but others will need to begin by holding both knees to their chests. Experiment to find which position feels best, and use that as your start position.

Beginning with knees to chest: Hold your right knee with both hands. Inhale, then exhale (draw your belly button in toward your spine) while you lower your left foot to the floor (your left knee should be bent at 90 degrees); stop if you feel back or pelvic pain or if you feel your back arch off the floor. Inhale, then raise your knee up again as you exhale while drawing your belly button toward your spine. Inhale, then exhale, and allow your right foot to slowly lower to the floor, with your knee bent at 90 degrees. Stop when you feel changes associated with losing the ideal spine position mentioned above. Inhale, then exhale to return back up. Repeat until you become fatigued, you experience lower back pain, or you can't control your spine. To progress this exercise, try not holding the opposite knee to your chest while lowering your leg. See if you have the strength to control your spine without using your arms to help. Gradually work toward a start position with both feet on the floor.

Beginning with both feet on floor: Draw your belly button in toward your spine and exhale while sliding your left foot away from you. Don't lift your leg off the floor. Stop if you feel back pain or feel your lower back arching up off the floor. To monitor this, put your fingers on either side of your lower spine to sense

COMMON ERRORS

• If your spine arches off the floor, you're performing the exercise too aggressively, or you aren't stabilizing adequately with your lower abdominal muscles. Slow down and develop better awareness of what your spine is doing. It's not a contest, so take it slow and do it right.

• If your neck arches, you're not stabilizing your lower spine well enough. Draw your belly button in toward your spine while flaring your ribs out. Stop if your neck arches.

• Rotation problems: If you have a rotated pelvis, you'll notice that one leg won't be able to drop down or slide out as far as the other leg before your spine begins to arch. Work within your ability, and do not allow your spine to arch even if you can't get your leg further out. Remember, your back pain is caused by a spine that arches too much or is rotated—and that should be your focus, not worrying about how far you can scoot out your leg.

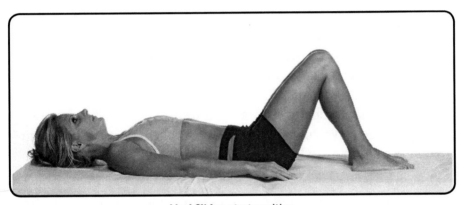

Heel Slides, start position

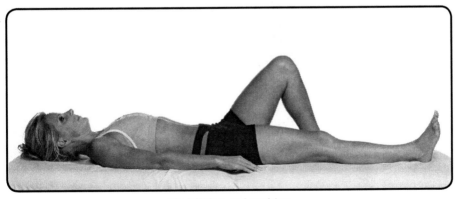

Heel Slides, end position

KNEE WOBBLES (FOR ROTATION PROBLEMS)

This exercise strengthens the abdominals' ability to stabilize against pelvic rotation. Your knees should be able to rotate out about 30–40 degrees without pelvic movement.

THE FIXING YOU METHOD

Lie on your back with knees bent, flattened lumbar spine, and hands on your hip bones (ASISs) to monitor their movement. The ASISs are the bony points that stick out in front of your pelvis. Engage your lower abdominals by drawing your belly button in toward your spine and/or exhaling by pushing your belly button toward your spine. Slowly lower your right knee out to the side; monitor your left ASIS for movement. Make sure your left ASIS doesn't rise up into your hand. Stop at the point where it rises. Inhale, then exhale while you try to lower your right knee further without left ASIS movement. If you find you can't keep that left ASIS from rising more, then return to the start position. Repeat on the opposite side. Always alternate sides to reestablish a pelvic baseline. If you continually work on the same side, then the opposite ASIS will gradually rise and you won't know it. If you notice that one side stays down more easily than the other, it could mean you have a rotated pelvis.

COMMON ERRORS

• If one ASIS comes up too soon, keep trying to stabilize using your abdominals. Don't allow your hip to come up, as this reinforces pelvic rotation.

• If you feel your ASIS stay down while you're lowering your leg to the side, but you feel it drop toward the floor when you return, then it's creeping up without your being aware. Develop your sensitivity to discern this movement.

• Don't stabilize your pelvis by pressing the opposite foot into the floor. Keep your leg relaxed; use your abdominals to stabilize instead.

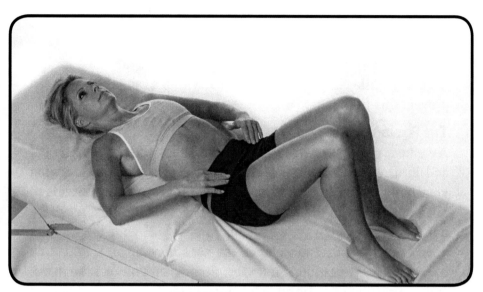

Knee Wobbles, start position

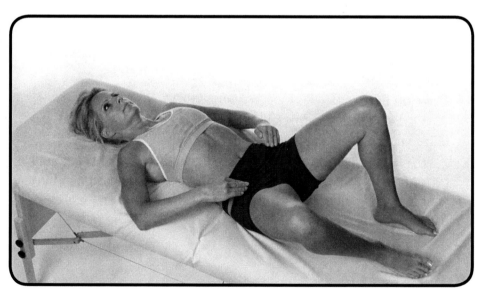

Knee Wobbles, end position

GLUTEAL PUMPS

This exercise restores strength to the **gluteus maximus**. This muscle often becomes weak, especially in the presence of tight muscles in the front of the pelvis. The hardest part of this exercise is keeping your spine from sagging down (increased lordotic curve) while exercising. Only work within a range that you can prevent this from happening.

THE FIXING YOU METHOD

Assume a position on your elbows and knees with your spine flat and in a neutral position. Hold your spine in place by drawing your belly button in toward your spine. Squeeze your **gluteals** to raise one leg up in the air with your knee bent at 90 degrees. Try not to push your leg up with your foot or pull your leg up with your hamstrings (the muscles in the back of your leg). Pull it up by squeezing your gluteal muscles. Stop when you feel the maximal contraction of these muscles. Slowly lower your leg about 1/4 to 1/2 inch. This ensures the glutes stay turned on and are doing the work. Maintain the gluteal contraction while you slowly pump your leg up and down. Make the gluteals fatigue. Perform 10–30 repetitions or until fatigue or failure (indicated if your hamstrings begin to fatigue instead of your gluteals). Switch sides.

COMMON ERRORS

• Don't arch your back to bring your leg up higher. Instead, stabilize your spine by drawing in your belly button.

• If your hamstrings cramp or fatigue, then you're using your hamstrings instead of your gluteals to lift your leg. Focus on pulling your leg up by squeezing your gluteus maximus (rear end muscles). Keep your hamstrings relatively relaxed.

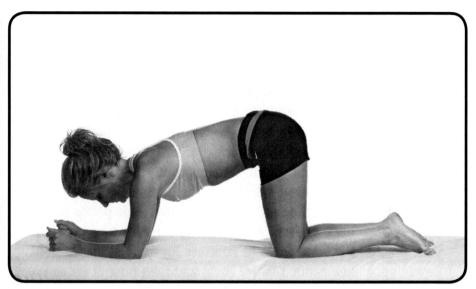

Gluteal Pumps, start position

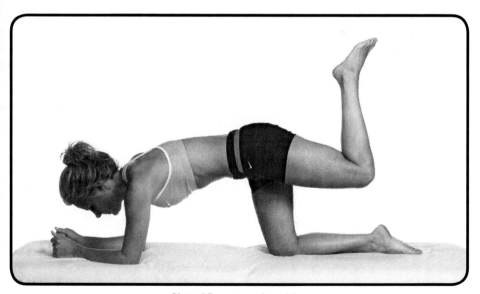

Gluteal Pumps, end position

SIDE-LYING CLAMSHELLS

This exercise restores strength to pelvic muscles that become stretched out and weak, which contributes to sciatic and pelvic pain. Keep the range of motion relatively small.

THE FIXING YOU METHOD

Lie on your left side with knees bent and spine in a neutral position. Stack your hip bones on top of each other. Exhale forcefully and/or draw your belly button in toward your spine to engage your abdominals and stabilize your spine and pelvis. Put your fingers on the back of your hip to monitor contraction of your muscles. Keep your top heel resting on the bottom heel, and raise your right knee to create an arc. Don't allow your pelvis to roll back or your back to arch. Feel your hip muscles turn on under your fingers. We want them to contract for as long as possible. Lower your knee about 1/4–1/2 inch, and then raise it up again. You should feel the muscles under your fingers working hard. Continue to raise your knee up and down while you maintain the contraction. Stop if back or hip pain occurs or you are unable to maintain good form. Perform 5–15 repetitions or until fatigued. Switch sides.

COMMON ERRORS

• Don't let your top hip rock back in order to raise your knee. This favors the TFL. Make the movement smaller, so your hip doesn't rock backward.

• If back or hip pain occurs, make sure the top heel is resting on the bottom heel. Try placing a towel or pillow between your knees. Limit the range of motion to a smaller range. Check to confirm your hips are stacked on top of each other.

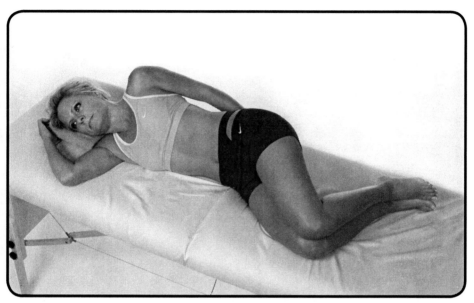

Side-Lying Clamshells, start position

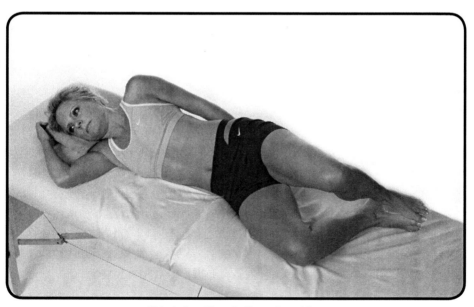

Side-Lying Clamshells, end position

FIXING YOU: BACK PAIN DURING PREGNANCY

GLOSSARY

abdominal muscles

Muscles on the anterior and lateral trunk that help to rotate and flex the spine. The abdominals are composed of several muscles.

rectus abdominus: Originates at the symphysis pubis and inserts into the sternum as well as the cartilage of ribs 5–7. This muscle flexes the spine and assists in posteriorly tilting the pelvis.

external obliques: One of the abdominal muscles responsible for rotation and flexion of the spine. Developing external oblique strength is important for spinal stabilization against movement dysfunctions.

internal obliques: One of the abdominal muscles responsible for rotation and flexion of the spine. Developing external oblique strength is important for spinal stabilization against movement dysfunctions.

transversus abdominus: An important spinal-stabilizing muscle.

anterior

In front of or forward. For instance, the toes are anterior to the heels.

anterior pelvic tilt

Occurs when the top of the pelvis tilts forward.

anterior superior illiac spine (ASIS)—See pelvis.

diastasis recti

Separation of the abdominal wall into left and right halves. If a separation of more than two fingers' width is present, a doctor visit is recommended to assess the integrity of the abdominal muscles.

extending

Regarding the spine, extending describes the movement wherein the spine bends backward from an upright position or returns from a flexed position.

extension

Describes a straightened joint position relative to a flexed position.

extension problem
A movement dysfunction wherein the spine is unable to flatten (flex) adequately or wherein the abdominals cannot stabilize the spine's extension, causing pain.

external obliques—See abdominal muscles.

flexing
The act of bending a joint. Bending forward or decreasing spinal extension involves flexing the spine.

flexion
Describes a flexed joint position relative to neutral or extension.

flexion problem
A movement dysfunction wherein the spine flexes too much or too soon at one or two vertebral levels or wherein the abdominals cannot stabilize the flexion of the spine, causing pain. Typically, this involves hips that do not flex well.

gluteals
A collective term for the gluteus maximus and gluteus medius.

gluteus maximus
This hip muscle runs from the ilium and sacrum to insert into the ITB and femur at the hip joint. Its actions include leg extension, external rotation, and guiding the femoral head in the hip socket.

gluteus medius
This hip muscle originates around the border of the anterior through posterior portions of the ilium and inserts onto the femur. The anterior fibers medially rotate the leg, the posterior fibers laterally rotate the leg and all working together abduct the leg.

hip
The joint where the femur and pelvis meet. This is a ball-and-socket joint, similar to the shoulder, that can move in many directions.

hyperextended joint
A joint that extends too far or too easily is said to be hyperextended.

hypermobile joint
A joint that has too much motion that may or may not be well controlled. A hypermobile joint often occurs near a hypomobile joint.

hypomobile joint
A joint that has too little motion. When a joint does not move well, other joints above or below it typically must compensate by becoming hypermobile in order to achieve functional movement.

impingement
Describes a condition wherein a tissue has become pinched or compressed, usually between two bones.

internal obliques—See abdominal muscles.

kyphosis
The natural outward curve of the thoracic spine; the opposite of lordosis.

linea alba
A tendinous line down the center of the abdominal muscles that divides them into left and right halves.

lordosis
The natural inward curve of the lumbar and cervical spine; the opposite of kyphosis.

lumbar vertebra—See vertebrae.

pelvis
The collection of bones on which our spine rests and with which our legs articulate. Pelvic position is important for spinal function. It is composed of several parts.

> **sacrum:** A series of fused vertebra that articulate with the lowest lumbar vertebra and both ilia, as well as the coccyx.

> **ilia (singular ilium):** Two irregularly shaped bones that articulate with the sacrum and house the hip socket where the femur articulates. Other landmarks of the ilium include:

> > **ASIS (anterior superior iliac spine):** A landmark to which the tensor fascia lata attaches and below which the rectus femoris attaches. This is an important landmark for assessing

pelvic rotation.

symphysis pubis: A joint formed by the pubic bones of both ilia. The orientation of the ASIS and symphysis pubis determines whether the pelvis is anteriorly or posteriorly rotated (see related terms).

iliac crest: The top edge of the ilium. Feeling the iliac crests and comparing them side to side helps form a more complete picture of the pelvis's contribution to back pain or hip pain.

posterior pelvic tilt

Occurs when the top of the pelvis tilts backward.

rectus abdominus—See abdominal muscles.

relaxin

A hormone believed to increase the pelvis's ability to loosen in preparation for birth.

rotation

A spinal movement whereby one vertebra rotates left or right in relation to another vertebra.

rotation problem

Term given to a spine that is more or less stuck in a rotated position to the right or left. Therefore, excessive rotation will occur in one direction and decreased rotation in the other.

sciatic nerve

A major nerve feeding the leg that originates in the lumbar vertebrae and travels down the back of the leg.

side-bending

A movement of the spine that ideally creates a lateral C-curve.

transversus abdominus (TA)—See abdominal muscles.

vertebrae (singular vertebra)

The bones that comprise the spine. They are divided into three sections.

cervical: The neck region. There are seven cervical vertebrae. They form an inward, lordotic curve.

thoracic: The upper trunk region where the ribs attach. There are twelve thoracic vertebrae. They form an outward, kyphotic curve.

lumbar: The lower spine region composed of five vertebrae. They form an inward, lordotic curve.

REFERENCES

Introduction opening quote:
Nechis, Barbara. 1993. *Watercolor from the Heart*. New York: Watson-Guptill Publications.

Section 1 opening quote:
Yogananda, Paramahansa. 1997. *Journey to Self-Realization*. Los Angeles, CA: Self-Realization Fellowship.

Section 2 opening quote:
Chopra, Deepak. 1993. *Creating Affluence: Wealth Consciousness in the Field of All Possibilities*. San Rafael, CA: New World Library.

Section 3 opening quote:
Campbell, Joseph. 1991. *The Joseph Campbell Companion: Reflections on the Art of Living*. Ed. Diane K. Osbon. New York: HarperCollins.

Kendall, Florence, Elizabeth McCreary, and Patricia Provance. 1993. *Muscles: Testing and Function, with Posture and Pain*. Fourth edition. Baltimore, MD: Williams & Wilkins.

Sahrmann, Shirley A. 2002. *Diagnosis and Treatment of Movement Impairment Syndromes*. St. Louis, MO: Mosby.

Rick Olderman MSPT, CPT

Following graduation in 1996 from the nationally ranked Krannert School of Physical Therapy at the University of Indianapolis, I practiced at a small sports and orthopedic clinic in Cortez, Colorado. Because the clinic had a small gym attached, I was able to progress patients to a higher functional level than if I were in a typical clinic. This unique model influenced me to consider personal training. I discovered that setting up therapeutic training programs for my patients helped them as much or more than any intervention I would perform manually.

I moved to Denver in 1999 and began working as a physical therapist and personal trainer at an exclusive health club, The Athletic Club at Denver Place. While there, I continued to experiment with blending rehabilitation and personal training and added Pilates to my skill set. Within just a few months, I became the top-producing employee at the club. I held that position for the next four years until I opened my own studio/clinic.

In addition to providing individual client services, I also lead corporate seminars for injury prevention and correction. My focus on teaching employees the fundamentals of injury mechanics and practical ways to correct them has made me an effective force in changing corporate thinking about injuries, injury prevention, ergonomics, and fitness programs. I believe education is the key. I find that if you teach someone how the body works and why they experience pain, most people will be more diligent in helping themselves. No one wants to be in pain.

I am an active member of the American Physical Therapy Association, and I continue to explore combined rehabilitation and fitness techniques through professional development and continuing education. I live and work in Denver, Colorado with my wife and two young children.

To access your free video demonstrations of all exercises in this book, visit **www.FixingYou.net**, select the Back Pain During Pregnancy book under the "Books" tab at the top, and then click the "View Video Clips" button. Once on the video clip page, type in the code: **abdominals**.

Lightning Source UK Ltd.
Milton Keynes UK
15 March 2011

169287UK00007B/75/P